Foreword

It gives me great pleasure to introduce this third edition of the A
First Aid at Work Training Organisations' course manual a
milestones. Firstly, with the printing of this edition, the Assoc
50,000 copies for its members. Second, year 2002 is the 10th y
Association. I was one of the first elected Executive Committee members and have enjoyed being part of its enormous growth. I have also been proud to be appointed its first President.

This manual symbolises the networking of well over 100 companies who have joined forces to work towards the maintaining of standards in First Aid training across the country and towards the mutual support of members. It has been produced by members of the Education Committee, whose aim is to try to ensure that the contents are clear, accurate and relevant to the needs of the workplace appointed person. The guidelines of HSE and the Resuscitation Councils have been closely followed.

As an appointed person you will hold a privileged and responsible position. Often working alone, your immediate actions will significantly affect the recovery of an ill or injured colleague. I hope you enjoy your training and wish you well in your future service as a valued appointed person in the workplace.

Muireall Lawson, RGN, OHNC

President

About this Manual

This manual is designed to accompany a structured course of learning in the practice of First Aid in the Workplace, in accordance with the Health and Safety (First Aid) Regulations 1992 and the accompanying Approved Code of Practice and Guidance. It does not profess to be exhaustive, or to be the only source of reference material which could accompany such training. However, it will serve as a good aid to revision during the course and a vital source of reference in the period following first aid qualification.

The content is based on the identified competencies for appointed person qualification, formulated and approved by the Association of Independent First Aid at Work Training Organisations.

It is unrealistic to expect a student to memorise all the text in this manual for assessment purposes. As an aid, the most important theory elements (underpinning knowledge) have been highlighted with a green background.

Delegate Name _____

Company _____

Course Dates _____

Index to Sections

Section	Title	Pages
1	First Aid at Work and the Law	1.1
2	Introduction to First Aid	2.1 - 2.5
3	Resuscitation	3.1 - 3.4
4	The Choking Casualty	4.1 - 4.3
5	Emergency Diagnosis	5.1 - 5.3
6	The Unconscious Casualty	6.1 - 6.7
7	Wounds and Bleeding	7.1 - 7.7
8	Shock	8.1 - 8.2
9	Head Injuries	9.1 - 9.2
10	General Illness at Work	10.1 - 10.2
11	Moving a Casualty	11.1 - 11.2
12	After an Accident at Work	12.1 - 12.2
13	First Aid Equipment	13.1 - 13.3

Appendix

I	Index to topics	I:1

First Aid at Work and the Law

Appointed Persons
HSC commission in their code of practice state that

Where an employer's assessment of first-aid needs identifies that a first aider is not necessary, the minimum requirement on an employer is to appoint a person to take charge of the first-aid arrangements, including looking after the equipment and facilities and calling the emergency services when required. Arrangements should be made for an appointed person to be available to undertake these duties at all times when people are at work.

Even in organisations with comparatively low health and safety risks where first aiders are considered unnecessary, there is always a possibility of accident or sudden illness. It is important, therefore, that someone is always available to take immediate action, such as calling an ambulance. Employers must, in the absence of first aiders, appoint a person for this purpose, though appointed persons are not necessary where there is an adequate number of first aiders.

It should be remembered that appointed persons are not first aiders and so should not attempt to give first aid for which they have not been trained. However, as the appointed person is required to look after the first-aid equipment and should ideally know how to use it, employers are strongly advised to consider the need for emergency first-aid training for appointed persons. Courses normally last four hours and cover the following topics:

- what to do in an emergency;
- cardio-pulmonary resuscitation;
- first aid for the unconscious casualty;
- first aid for the wounded or bleeding.

HSE approval is not required for this training.

The Regulations provide for a person to be appointed to provide emergency cover in the absence of first aiders by only where the absence is due to exceptional, unforeseen and temporary circumstances. Absence such as annual leave do not count. Remember that if the assessment calls for first aiders to be provided, they should be available whenever the need arises.

Introduction to First Aid

Before the practice of first aid can begin, it is essential that knowledge relating to the role and responsibilities of the appointed person are understood

The Responsibilities of an Appointed Person

There are five main responsibilities which face an appointed person in the workplace:

- Assess
- Diagnose
- Treat
- Dispose
- Record

Assess

On arrival at the scene of an accident, it is essential that a quick but thorough assessment is made relating to many factors:

1. **What happened?**

   Quickly determine the nature and circumstances of the accident.

2. **Is the area safe?**

   Assess the area for any danger which may be present. If the situation dictates that there is further danger to the appointed person or casualty then there are three courses of action to consider:

   a. Stay away.

   If the danger is extreme or beyond the appointed person's ability to cope, the best course of action is to keep well clear and leave the situation to qualified professional help. Do not become a casualty yourself!

   b. Move the danger.

   In some situations it may be possible to remove or isolate the danger at the scene of an accident, e.g. to turn off an electricity supply or to move an object which presents a falling or trip hazard. This method of dealing with danger is often the best as it does not involve moving the casualty from the scene, which could potentially make the casualty's condition worse.

   c. Move the casualty.

   In some situations it may be very difficult or impossible to remove or neutralise danger at the scene of an accident. If this is so, it may be necessary to remove the casualty from the source of danger. When this course of action is taken, try to minimise the risk of causing any further injury to the casualty by moving them carefully and, where possible, utilising the help of bystanders.

3. **How many casualties are there?**

   The accident may have given rise to several different casualties. If the history of the accident indicates that multiple casualties are possible, a quick sweep around the area should be undertaken to ensure all injured persons are accounted for. It may be possible to ask bystanders or casualties how many people were present at the accident area.

4. **Do I need help?**

   In some cases, the nature and magnitude of the incident may dictate that immediate help in the local vicinity is required. In many cases there may be bystanders who can help but in circumstances where the appointed person is alone it may be necessary to shout for help. When the appointed person is making their initial assessment at the scene of an accident it is very important that they remain calm and collected and do not add to any panic or confusion which may already be evident. It is often a good idea to introduce yourself as an appointed person as you arrive on the scene as this can help instil confidence and co-operation in others.

Diagnose

Before any definitive treatment can be given to a

casualty it is essential to evaluate their condition. This is called a diagnosis. There are three elements to consider when forming a diagnosis:

1. **History**

   This means how and when the accident or illness occurred. In some cases the cause and nature of the accident may be obvious but in some cases it may not. Bystanders at the scene of an accident may be able to tell you what happened or may even be able to tell you of any underlying medical condition from which the casualty is suffering. Clues may be evident which point toward a particular cause of injury or illness. Information regarding the cause and circumstances of the accident can be of considerable help in finding and diagnosing a casualty's condition. Think back to when you have been examined by a G.P. or casualty department doctor and the odds are that the first question they asked you was "How did you do this?"

   Things to look for include:
   - History of impact or violence to the casualty.
   - Evidence of electrocution or contact with a chemical substance.
   - Machinery or tools which the casualty may have been using.
   - Evidence of smoke or other harmful substances.
   - The history of an accident can give a very good indication as to the nature and severity of injuries which a casualty has sustained.

2. **Signs**

   All injuries and illnesses have particular pointers or features which may help with the diagnosis. Signs of injury or illness are the features discovered by applying four of your five senses when examining the casualty.

   a. Look:

   At the site of injury for swelling, deformity, unusual movement, bruising, foreign bodies, bleeding. At the casualty in general for anxiety or stress, painful expression, sweating, difficult or laboured breathing, abnormal skin colour, incontinence, injection/sting/bite marks, vomiting, any other signs of injury.

   b. Listen:

   For any unusual breathing sounds, to the legibility and clarity of the casualty's speech, to any statements made by the casualty or bystanders.

   c. Feel:

   For deformity of the bone structure, dampness in the groin region, skin temperature, tenderness, swelling.

   d. Smell:

   The casualty's breath for acetone (sweet smell) or alcohol.

3. **Symptoms**

   These are the sensations and feelings which the casualty has or may be able to describe to you. For example, the exact location of pain, weakness or paralysis, temperature and dizziness. You may need to ask questions to establish the presence or absence of some symptoms.

Useful questions for questioning a conscious casualty:

Q - What happened?

Is the response clear? Confused? Incomprehensible?

Q - What is your name?

Is the response clear? Confused? Incomprehensible?

Q - Exactly where is the pain?

Is the casualty capable of moving by themselves to indicate the area?

Q - Are you taking any medication or being seen by a doctor for any medical condition?

Q - Have you ever had this problem before? (In cases of suspected medical conditions.)

If yes, when? How often? Is it worse than last time?

Q - Are you allergic to anything?

Q - Is there anyone else I should inform about your condition? e.g. relative, work.

Remember :

HISTORY + SIGNS + SYMPTOMS = DIAGNOSIS

Treat

> The main aims of first-aid treatment for any injury or medical condition are to :
> - Save life.
> - Prevent the condition from becoming worse.

1. To Save Life

Knowing that your skills could save another person's life is a great incentive for learning. Even in a very hazardous working environment, situations where a person's life is at risk are not commonplace; indeed, the vast majority of appointed persons may never deal with anything more serious than a broken ankle or a small cut. This statistic, however, does not mean that an appointed person should ignore the possibility (no matter how remote) that they may at some time have to provide life saving treatments. Being prepared for the worst is very important.

2. To Prevent the Condition Becoming Worse

When a person is injured or ill, their condition can be classified into one of three possible states. It could be deteriorating (getting worse), stabilised (remaining constant) or improving (getting better). If the appointed person can stop, or at least slow down, the speed of deterioration in the casualty's condition, it could give the casualty a few more precious minutes which could mean the difference between life or death. This idea is best demonstrated by means of a graph.

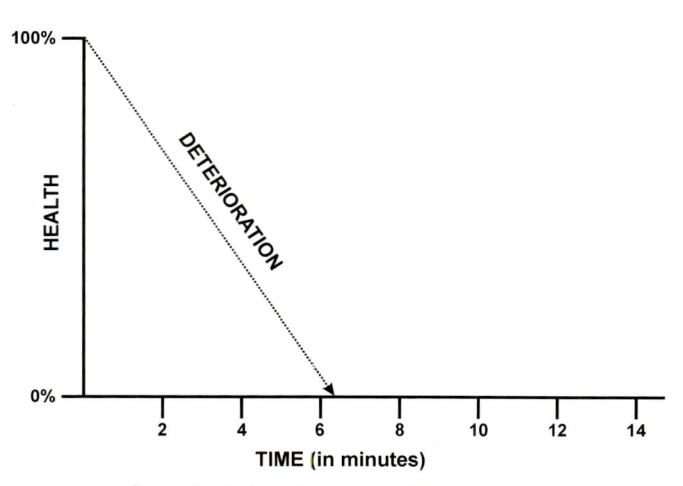

GRAPH 1 - Without Treatment

The first graph represents the conditional status of a casualty who is bleeding from a major open wound. It shows that without treatment the casualty will continue to deteriorate and eventually reach 0% health (or death) in six minutes.

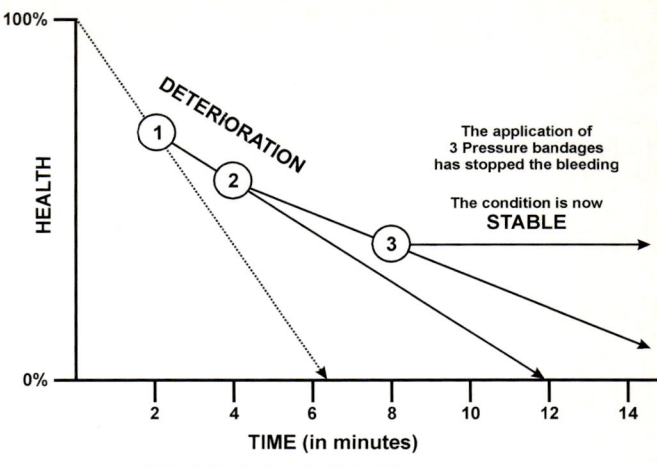

GRAPH 2 - With Treatment

The application of 3 Pressure bandages has stopped the bleeding

The condition is now **STABLE**

The second graph shows that at 2 minutes the casualty received some treatment for the bleeding (in this case the application of a pressure bandage over the wound) and this has an immediate effect. Although the casualty is still deteriorating, the speed of deterioration is less. Good observation of the casualty shows that by 4 minutes blood has seeped through the initial dressing so a second pressure dressing has been applied on top of the first. This extra pressure has slowed the bleeding down even further. Once again, good observation shows that by 8 minutes blood has seeped through the second dressing so a third pressure dressing is applied directly over the top of the second. Although still very serious, the casualty's condition is now stable. Overall conclusion - without treatment the casualty will die within 6 minutes, with treatment the casualty will still be alive when the emergency medical aid arrives.

Good first aid can, in some cases, actually result in a slight improvement of the casualty's condition although full recovery may take weeks or even years, depending on the nature and severity of the problem. There are some casualties for whom first aid is of little benefit, simply because their injury or condition is so severe. Even so, an appointed person should always do their best regardless of how pointless the task appears. There have been many cases where even qualified doctors have given a patient little or no hope of survival only to be proved wrong!

In some cases, the only treatment an appointed person in the workplace can give is simple advice to the casualty. Take, for example, a casualty who complains of toothache. There is no specific treatment for this condition and in most circumstances all the appointed person can do is offer advice to the casualty to the effect of "If the pain persists or gets worse, go see your dentist". Although no physical treatment has taken place, the fact that a person reported to the appointed person with a problem should still be recorded, alongside any advice that the appointed person gave. Who knows, maybe frequent aches and pains (including headaches) are the result of an environmental problem which secretly exists in the workplace? If all details are recorded, the company health and safety manager can identify the problem and, if necessary, investigate possible causes within the workplace.

In some instances, the appointed person may have to deal with more than one casualty or a single casualty with more than one injury. If this is the case it is important that treatments are prioritised, thus ensuring that the most serious injuries and conditions are treated first, and leaving minor injuries and conditions until last.

A basic but highly endorsed system of prioritisation is known as the A.B.C system.

Life threatening injuries and conditions should be prioritised in the following order:

1st **Airway.** Any condition which causes blockage or obstruction to the main breathing tubes of the respiratory system, particularly the mouth and throat.

2nd **Breathing.** Any condition which causes stoppage or interference with the mechanism of breathing.

3rd **Circulation.** Any condition which causes stoppage or interference with the circulation of blood around the body.

Non-life-threatening injuries and conditions should be prioritised in the following order:

1st Those likely to result in the deterioration of a casualty's condition, possibly to a life-threatening extent before the arrival of further medical aid.

2nd Those likely to result in no deterioration of a casualty's condition.

Dispose

This means the course of action to be taken after treatment by the appointed person. There are many potential methods of casualty disposal which an appointed person may consider:

1. Return to Work

In the majority of cases following minor injury, a casualty may return to work after treatment. If this is the case, however, the casualty should always be advised to report back to the appointed person or their doctor if the condition appears to worsen. A good example of this is a small 'paper cut'. Having received treatment by the appointed person, it may be that throughout the day the cut still bleeds slightly or, over the next few days, perhaps becomes infected. A good appointed person should always think carefully about the potential long term development of further problems arising with the condition (this is referred to as the prognosis) and advise the casualty accordingly. As already mentioned, the advice given to the casualty should also be recorded alongside any physical treatments which were given.

2. To see their own or company doctor

Some casualties may need to see a doctor shortly after injury or sudden illness even though the condition does not constitute an emergency. A good example of this is where a casualty has sustained a small open wound which is particularly dirty and fresh water alone is not adequate to deal with the potential infection (or perhaps the casualty may need a tetanus injection). Cleaning of wounds with antiseptic solutions or creams is well beyond the normal scope of first aid in the workplace and therefore, unless specifically trained and deemed competent, an appointed person should not attempt to use any medications to clean wounds. (Solutions and creams can also cause allergic reactions.) This is the responsibility of the casualty's own doctor's surgery, or if available, their company's Occupational Health department or nurse. If a visit to their own doctor is difficult at short notice, the casualty department of the local hospital should be considered, although treatment of this type of problem will take a very low priority.

3. Taken to Hospital (Non-emergency)

Although again not an emergency, a casualty's condition may often warrant further investigation and treatment from the casualty department of the local hospital. An example of this is a suspected broken hand or fingers. First-aid treatment can often be sufficient to stabilise the injury short term but the casualty will certainly need to be seen at hospital. Taken to hospital means exactly that - the casualty is escorted all the way, not just told to make their own way. Just imagine the consequences if a person with broken fingers tried to drive themselves to hospital!

4. Taken to Hospital (Emergency)

The only way that a casualty should be taken to hospital in an emergency situation is by an ambulance.

When calling for an ambulance the following information should be given in a clear, unhurried and logical sequence:

a. Confirmation of the telephone number from which the call is being made.
b. The name of the caller.
c. The exact location of the incident.
d. The nature or cause of the incident.
e. How many casualties there are and information relating to their general diagnosis.
f. What first aid treatments have already been administered.

The operator may ask other questions relating to the incident so it is important that the person making the call is familiar with the incident. When all information is passed, the operator may give an indication as to how long the ambulance may take to arrive. When finished, the operator should be the one to terminate the call.

If a bystander is used to make the call, it may be necessary for them to write down certain details to ensure that the information given is correct and the bystander should be told to report back to the appointed person when the call has been made.

In all cases where an emergency ambulance has been called to the workplace, the appointed person should ensure that their supervisor or line manager is informed of the occurrence at the earliest possible opportunity.

In many cases, the ambulance service may be able to give the appointed person further advice regarding the treatment and disposal of the casualty.

Record

All accidents in the workplace (even those where nobody was injured) have to be recorded in the accident book.

Test Your Knowledge

1) You are on your own and arrive at the scene of an accident involving 3 casualties:

   a) one person lying down, sobbing and obviously in severe pain
   b) one person who is sitting and is bleeding from a wound to the forearm
   c) one person with no obvious injuries who is lying face up and unconscious

   State which order you should prioritise these: a) .... b) .... c) ....

2) In order to be able to survive, a person must have:

   i   A.....................................
   ii B.....................................
   iii C.....................................

3) The first and most important thing you should do on arrival at the scene of an accident is to (please tick one answer):

   a) check the airway of the casualty   b) check for dangers
   c) phone for an ambulance   d) control severe bleeding

Resuscitation

The ability to take over for another person's breathing and circulation by artificial means are essential skills for all appointed persons.

Resuscitation is the act of restoring function to the circulatory and/or respiratory systems when, for whatever reason, they have stopped.

Reasons why a person's breathing and circulation may stop are numerous, but the most common reasons include:

- Heart attack.
- Electric shock.
- Head injury.
- Poisoning, including drugs.
- Drowning.
- Blood loss leading to shock.

Stoppage of breathing and circulation is very serious, and quick diagnosis and treatment is essential.

Stoppage of Breathing

Stoppage of breathing is often referred to as respiratory arrest.

Diagnosis

Carry out the emergency diagnosis procedure (see section 7).

- Assess **Danger** (ensure safety).
- Assess **Response** (gently shake the casualty and shout for help in the local vicinity).
- Assess **Airway** (head tilt - chin lift).
- Assess **Breathing** (look, listen and feel).
- Assess **Circulation**.

Artificial Ventilation (Rescue Breathing).

If the casualty is not breathing normally, it is necessary to supply their body with oxygen by artificially ventilating their lungs (rescue breathing). The commonest form of rescue breathing used by appointed persons is called mouth-to-mouth ventilation.

- If a bystander is available at the scene, send them for an ambulance as soon as you know that the casualty is not breathing.

- Turn the casualty onto their back if they are not already in this position.

- Give two effective breaths of mouth-to-mouth ventilation, each of which makes the chest rise:

  - Ensure head tilt. Remove any visible obstruction from the casualty's mouth including dislodged dentures, but leave well-fitting dentures in place. Lift the chin.

    Pinch the soft part of the casualty's nose closed with the index finger and thumb of the hand which is on their forehead.

  - Open the casualty's mouth a little but maintain chin lift. Take a deep breath and place your lips around their mouth, making sure that you have a good seal.

  - Blow steadily into their mouth over about 1 to 2 seconds, watching for their chest rising, as in normal breathing (in an adult, this usually requires 700-1000 ml of air). Be careful not to over-inflate the lungs as this may cause more problems.

  - Maintaining head tilt and chin lift, take your mouth away from the casualty and watch for their chest to fall as the air comes out.

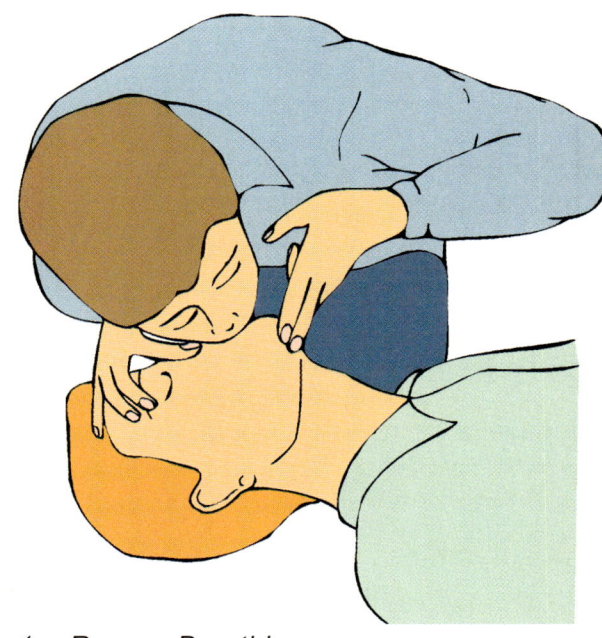

Fig.1. Rescue Breathing

  - Take another breath and repeat the sequence.

  - If you have difficulty in achieving an effective breath:

- Re-check the casualty's mouth and remove any visible obstruction.
- Re-check that there is adequate head tilt and chin lift.
- Make up to five attempts in all to achieve two effective breaths.

Even if unsuccessful, move on to assessment of circulation.

● Assess **Circulation**

(Assessment of the carotid pulse is time-consuming and often unrealiable. Performing a pulse check as a sign of cardiac arrest is no longer recommended for lay first-aiders.)

Look, listen and feel for normal breathing, coughing, or movement by the victim.

Take no more than 10 seconds to do this.

● If you are confident that you can detect signs of circulation within 10 seconds:

Continue rescue breathing, at a rate of one breath every six seconds, if necessary, until the casualty starts breathing on their own.

About every 10 breaths (or every one minute) recheck for signs of circulation. Take no more than 10 seconds each time.

● If the casualty begins to breathe normally on their own but remains unconscious, treat as for the unconscious casualty (see section 9).

● If there are no signs of circulation or if you are at all unsure, start chest compressions.

(Health care providers should still perform a pulse check as a sign of cardiac arrest and appointed persons can still use a pulse check for monitoring the condition of an unconscious casualty as part of a top-to-toe survey.)

Stoppage of Circulation

Stoppage of circulation is often referred to as cardiac arrest. In cases of cardiac arrest, it is necessary to provide artificial circulation of the casualty's blood. The commonest method of providing artificial circulation is called chest compressions.

This is a very physical procedure in which firm pressure is applied to the casualty's chest with the intention of compressing the heart and pumping blood around the body.

Chest Compressions

● Locate the lower half of the casualty's breastbone (sternum):

- Using your index and middle fingers, identify the lower rib margin. Keeping your fingers together, slide them upwards to the point where the ribs join the sternum. With the middle finger on this point, place your index finger on the sternum.
- Slide the heel of your other hand down the sternum until it reaches your index finger; this should be the middle of the lower half of the sternum.
- Place the heel of the other hand on top of the first.
- Interlock the fingers of both hands and lift them to ensure that pressure is not applied to the casualty's ribs. Do not apply any pressure over the upper abdomen or bottom tip of the sternum.

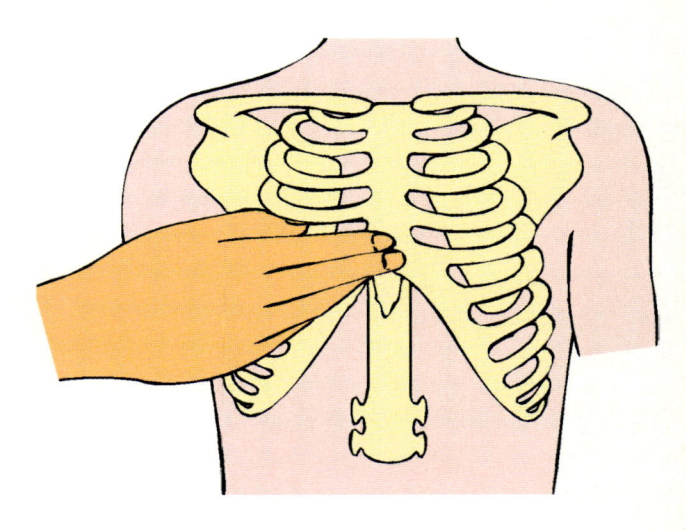

Fig. 2. Compression Point

● Position yourself vertically above the casualty's chest and with your arms straight, press down on the sternum to depress it between 4-5cm (1½ to 2 inches).

Interlock fingers.

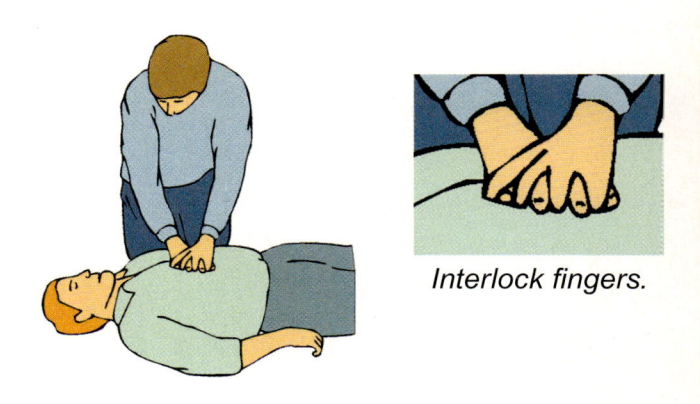

Fig. 3. Performing Chest Compressions

- Release the pressure, without losing contact between the hand and sternum, then repeat at a rate of 100 times a minute (a little less than two compressions a second). Compression and release should take an equal amount of time.

- Combine rescue breathing and chest compression:
  - After 15 compressions, tilt the head, lift the chin and give two effective breaths.

    Return your hands without delay to the correct position on the sternum and give 15 further compressions, continuing breaths and compressions at a ratio of 2 to 15.

- Continue resuscitation until:
  - The ambulance arrives.
  - You become exhausted.
  - The casualty shows signs of life.

Only stop to recheck for signs of a circulation if the victim makes a movement or takes a spontaneous breath; otherwise, resuscitation should not be interrupted. If the casualty should at any point show signs of life or a return of circulation, eg movement, breathing, swallowing, coughing, etc, reassess for signs of a circulation. If you are confident that you can detect signs of circulation, stop performing chest compressions and continue rescue breathing at a rate of one ventilation every six seconds and re-check circulation every one minute.

As HSE recommends that any appointed person working regularly alone has the means to summon help in an emergency, it is unlikely that an appointed person should need to leave any casualty.

When Do I Call for an Ambulance?

It is essential that professional help is called quickly if a casualty is not breathing. Therefore, if there is a bystander or helper at the scene, send them to call for an ambulance as soon as you know that the casualty is unresponsive and is not breathing.

If you are alone and the casualty is not breathing:

- If the likely cause of unconsciousness is,

  Alcohol or
  Drug intoxication;
  Drowning; or if it is an
  Infant or child; or
  Choking; or
  Trauma

  give the two breaths of artificial ventilation and assess for signs of circulation (as above). Resuscitate the casualty with artificial ventilation and if appropriate with chest compressions for one minute, then leave the casualty to call for help. On return to the casualty, recheck A.B.C. and continue resuscitation as necessary.

- If the likely cause of unconsciousness is as above, the appointed person should assume that the casualty has a heart problem and go for help immediately it has been established that the casualty is not breathing. On return to the casualty, recheck A.B.C. and begin resuscitation as necessary.

Test Your Knowledge

1) You are attending an adult casualty who has just collapsed in front of you. There are no injuries. You find that they are not breathing and have no pulse. You are on your own. What immediate action should you take (please tick one answer):

    a) Leave the casualty and 'phone for an ambulance before commencing resuscitation.
    b) Commence resuscitation for a minute before 'phoning for an ambulance.
    c) Carry out resuscitation until help arrives.
    d) Place them into the recovery position and wait for someone else to arrive.

2) You are dealing with an unconscious adult casualty who has just been struck on the head by a falling scaffold pole. After checking that the airway is clear and open, you find that he is not breathing. You are on your own. What immediate action will you take (please tick one answer):

    a) Leave the casualty and 'phone for an ambulance before commencing resuscitation.
    b) Commence resuscitation for a minute before 'phoning for an ambulance.
    c) Carry out resuscitation until help arrives.
    d) Place them into the recovery position and wait for someone else to arrive.

3) How would you decide whether a casualty had stopped breathing?

    a) ....   b) ....   c) ....

4) How would you resuscitate someone who was bleeding from the mouth?

    ....

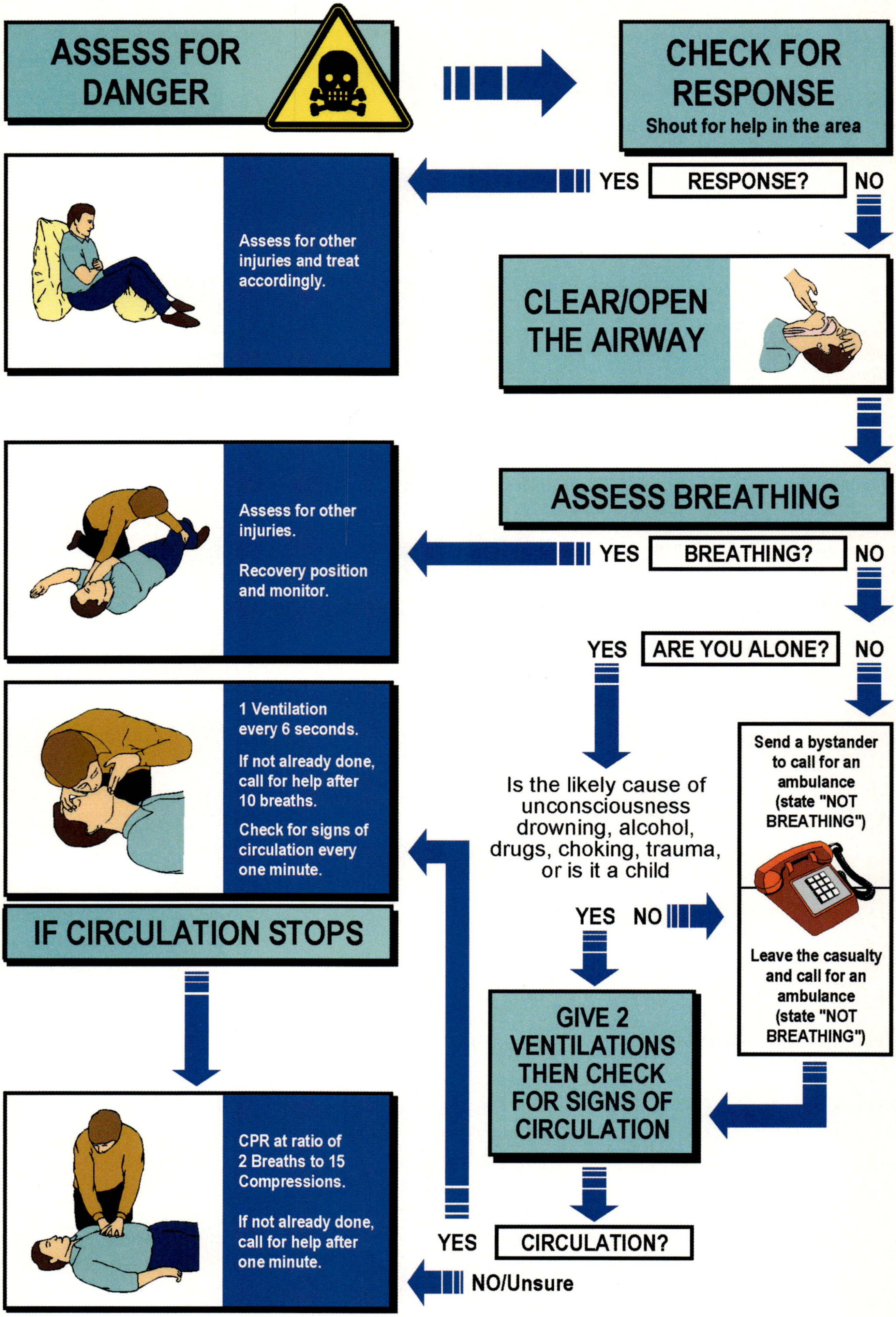

SECTION 3 — APPOINTED PERSON'S MANUAL

ASSESS FOR DANGER

CHECK FOR RESPONSE
Shout for help in the area

RESPONSE?
- YES → Assess for other injuries and treat accordingly.
- NO ↓

CLEAR/OPEN THE AIRWAY

ASSESS BREATHING

BREATHING?
- YES → Assess for other injuries. Recovery position and monitor.
- NO ↓

ARE YOU ALONE?
- YES ↓
- NO → Send a bystander to call for an ambulance (state "NOT BREATHING")

Is the likely cause of unconsciousness drowning, alcohol, drugs, choking, trauma, or is it a child
- YES ↓
- NO → Leave the casualty and call for an ambulance (state "NOT BREATHING")

GIVE 2 VENTILATIONS THEN CHECK FOR SIGNS OF CIRCULATION

CIRCULATION?
- YES → 1 Ventilation every 6 seconds. If not already done, call for help after 10 breaths. Check for signs of circulation every one minute.
- NO/Unsure ↓

IF CIRCULATION STOPS

CPR at ratio of 2 Breaths to 15 Compressions.

If not already done, call for help after one minute.

Fig.4. Resuscitation Flow Chart

The Choking Casualty

Airway obstruction is a very common cause of asphyxia and death. It is therefore essential that it can be recognised and treated quickly.

The Conscious Choking Casualty

Lying behind the larynx is another tube which passes down through the neck. This is the oesophagus down which food and drink pass to the stomach. The upper aspect of the oesophagus opens out into the back of the throat just behind the top of the windpipe. One tube should carry only gas and the other should carry only solid and liquid but with the close proximity of the two tube openings there is a potential for error. To overcome this problem there is a small flap of cartilage and soft tissue located above the opening of the windpipe called the epiglottis. When we swallow the neck muscles contract and this moves the epiglottis over the top of the windpipe, sealing it off. This ensures that the swallowed substance can only pass down one of the two tubes - the oesophagus.

The swallowing reflex, although simple in design, requires a great deal of muscular co-ordination. If the co-ordination is not precise, it results in incorrect positioning of the epiglottis during the swallowing process. Therefore, when the swallowed substance reaches the back of the throat, the top of the windpipe will be slightly open and the substance will enter the air passage (it's gone down the wrong hole).

The passage of a solid or liquid substance into the top of the windpipe causes a massive and quite dramatic response. Firstly, the neck muscles go into involuntary spasm. Second, the cough reflex will often try to expel the object.

Recognition

- The casualty may panic and become distressed.
- If standing, the casualty may stagger, become unsteady on their feet and may collapse.
- In the early stages the casualty's face may become flushed. In the later stages it may become pale, and cyanosis (blueness) may develop at the extremities.
- The casualty will be making distressed and perhaps violent efforts to breathe.
- The casualty's hands may grasp for the throat.
- The casualty's eyes may stare and begin to bulge.
- The casualty will often adopt a forward leaning posture. This helps the abdominal muscles to contract thus increasing the power of the cough reflex.

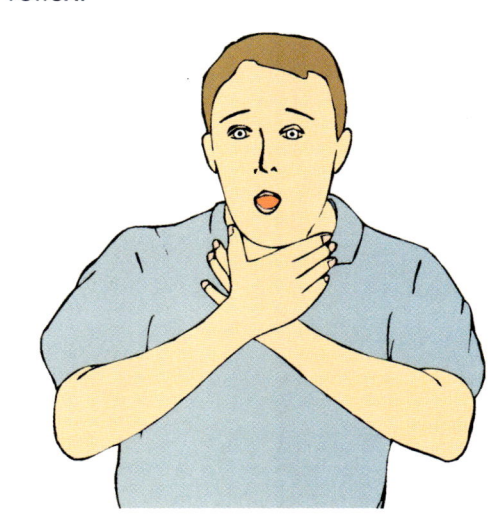

Fig.5. The Choking Casualty

Treatment

A situation where a person is choking can be very distressing for all concerned, but it is very important that treatment is administered in a calm and reassuring manner.

- If you are unaware of the history of the situation, ask the casualty if they are choking. They may confirm your suspicion with a nod.
- If possible, keep the casualty still (sitting or standing).
- Loosen any obvious tight, restrictive clothing such as a neck tie or belt.
- If the casualty is breathing, encourage him to continue coughing but do nothing else.
- If the casualty shows signs of becoming weak or stops breathing or coughing, leave him in the position in which you find him, remove any obvious debris or loose false teeth from the

mouth and carry out **back slaps.**

- Stand behind or to the side of the casualty, keeping them leaning well forward.
- Using the heel of the hand, give up to 5 sharp slaps between their shoulder blades.

Each slap may relieve the obstruction and it may not be necessary to give all five.

During the process, watch carefully for the object being expelled onto the floor.

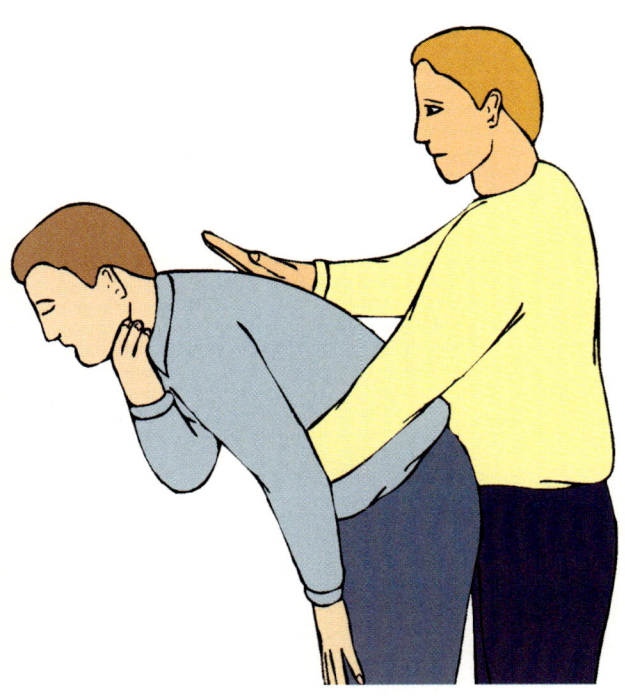

Fig.6. Administering Back Slaps

- If back slaps fail, **abdominal thrusts** may be tried.

The abdominal thrust is a very physical procedure to perform on a casualty and due to possible complications it should not be carried out on heavily pregnant women or on infants (see appendix H).

- Stand behind the casualty and put your arms around the casualty. Make a fist with one hand and place it against the casualty's upper abdomen (between the bottom of the breastbone and the navel) with the thumb innermost. Grasp the fist with the other hand.
- Pull sharply inwards and upwards. This has the effect of pushing the diaphragm upward and compressing the lungs. The obstruction should be expelled just like a cork from a bottle.

This abdominal thrust procedure may be attempted up to five times.

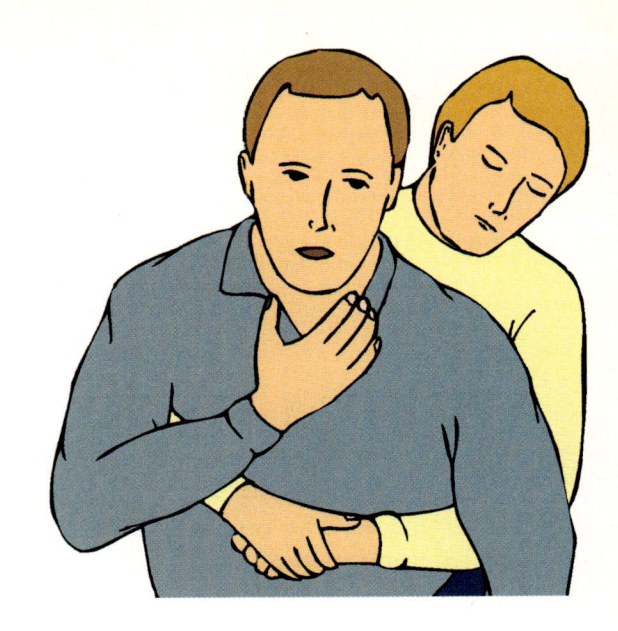

Fig.7. Administering Abdominal Thrusts

- If the obstruction is still not removed re-check the mouth for any obstruction which can be reached with a finger and continue alternating between five back slaps and five abdominal thrusts until either the object is removed or the casualty becomes unconscious.
- If the object is removed, put the casualty at rest and reassure them. Stay with the casualty and monitor them until breathing and skin colour return to normal.
- Any casualty on whom the abdominal thrust has been performed should be taken to hospital for further examination.

If the throat of any casualty who has been choking remains sore, or shows any evidence of damage or bleeding, they should be taken to hospital for further examination.

To sum up choking for a conscious casualty:

- encourage to cough.
- give 5 back slaps.
- give 5 abdominal thrusts.
- repeat 5 slaps and 5 thrusts as necessary.

The Unconscious Choking Casualty

If the object is not removed from the throat, it may lead to unconsciousness.

Unconsciousness may result in relaxation of the muscles around the larynx (voicebox) and allow air to pass down into the lungs:

- Call for an ambulance.
- Carry out ABC and try to give 2 effective rescue breaths.

● continue chest compressions and/or rescue breaths, as appropriate.

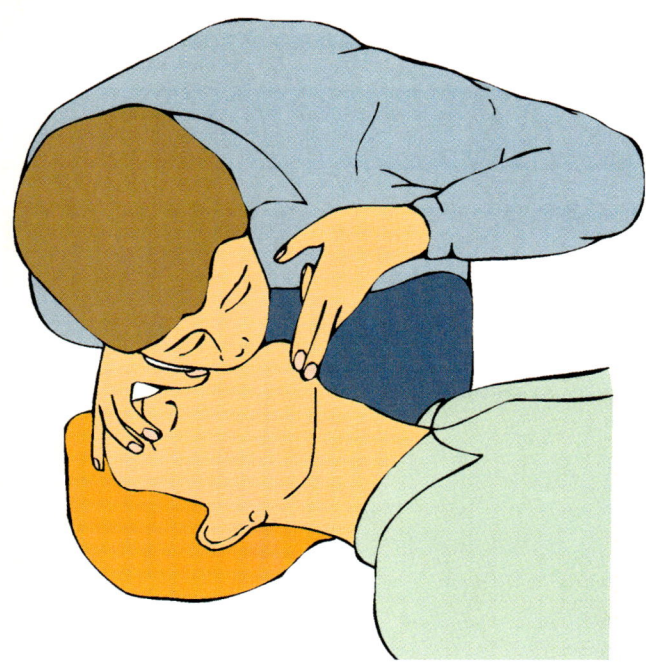

Fig.8. Rescue Breaths – Unconscious Choking Casualty

● If effective breaths **can** be achieved within 5 attempts, check for signs of a circulation (section 7) and start chest compressions and/or rescue breaths, as appropriate.

● If effective breaths **cannot** be achieved within 5 attempts, start chest compressions **immediately** to relieve the obstruction – do not check for signs of a circulation (it wastes time).

● After 15 compressions, check the mouth for any obstruction and then attempt further rescue breaths.

Continue to give cycles of 15 compressions followed by attempts at rescue breaths. If at any time effective breaths **can** be achieved:

● check for signs of a circulation.

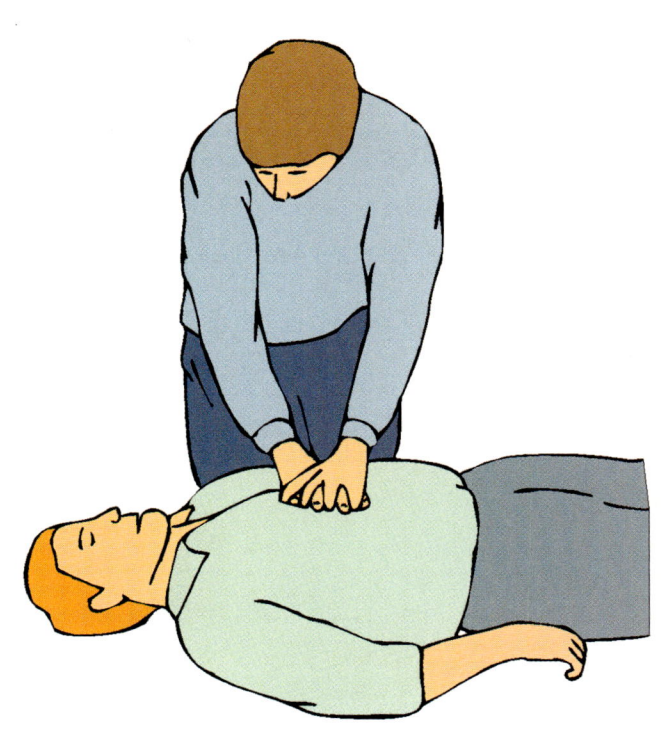

Fig.9. Chest Compressions – Unconscious Choking Casualty

To sum up choking for an unconscious casualty:
● carry out A and B of ABC.
● if breaths achieved, do C of ABC.
● do chest compressions or rescue breaths, as appropriate.
● if breaths not achieved, do NOT do C of ABC.
● do 15 compressions and 2 breaths.
● repeat as necessary.

Test Your Knowledge

1) What is the correct sequence for someone who has food stuck in his throat (please tick one):

    a) encourage to cough, 5 backslaps between shoulder blades, 5 abdominal thrusts
    b) 5 backslaps between shoulder blades, encourage to cough, 5 abdominal thrusts
    c) 5 backslaps between shoulder blades, 5 abdominal thrusts, encourage to cough
    d) 5 abdominal thrusts, encourage to cough, 5 backslaps between shoulder blades

2) What may prevent air getting through to the casualty's lungs during mouth-to-mouth?
    ....

3) If someone is choking and becomes unconscious and non-breathing, is it worth giving rescue breaths? ....

    Give a reason for your answer..

Emergency Diagnosis

Assessing the general condition of a casualty is the cornerstone of effective management. Incorrect diagnosis leads to incorrect treatment.

Before any treatment can commence, a diagnosis must be made to ascertain the general condition of the casualty. It is essential (and logical) that the most life-threatening conditions are found and treated first.

If the condition of a conscious casualty deteriorates, they will eventually become unconscious which causes voluntary muscles in the body to relax.

If an already unconscious casualty continues to deteriorate, the involuntary muscles of the body will stop working. Involuntary muscles are controlled subconsciously, that is to say a person does not have to think about their movement for the movement to occur. Examples of involuntary muscles are the diaphragm and the heart muscle. Just imagine how difficult life would be if you had to consciously think about it for your breathing and heart beat to occur!

The first group of involuntary muscles to stop functioning after unconsciousness are those concerned with breathing, i.e. the diaphragm and the intercostals. Stoppage of breathing is referred to as Respiratory Arrest.

If a non-breathing casualty should continue to deteriorate, the next group of involuntary muscles which will stop working are those of the heart. Stoppage of the heart is referred to as Cardiac Arrest.

The graph shows the possible path of deterioration of a casualty from 100% health down to death. As you can see, it is only a matter of minutes before unconsciousness, respiratory and cardiac arrest occur.

Every casualty who an appointed person would need to treat will fall into one of the four different diagnosis areas or zones. Emergency Diagnosis is the procedure undertaken to ascertain which zone a casualty is presently in.

In this graph format, it is easy to see that generally a zone 2 casualty is worse than a zone 1 casualty. A zone 3 is worse than a zone 2 and so on. The worst possible general condition a casualty can be in, regardless of cause, is cardiac arrest.

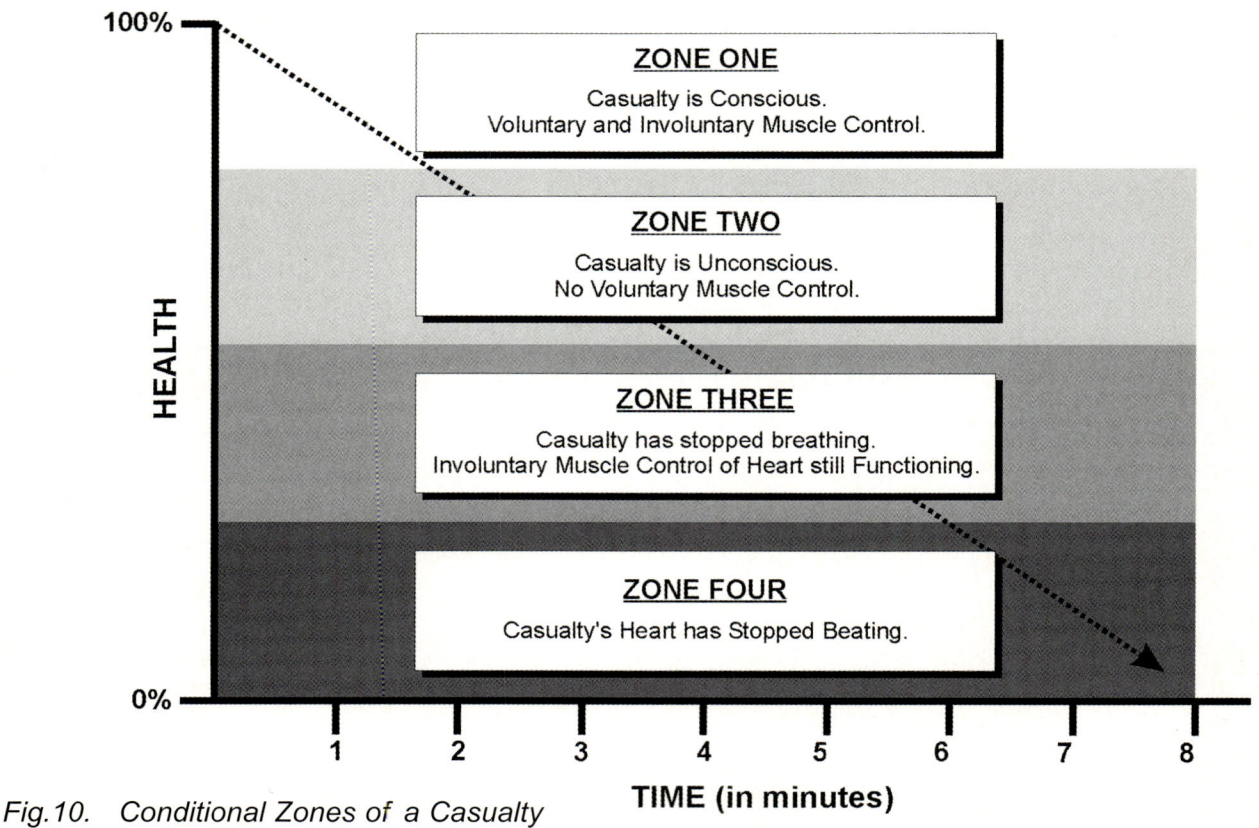

ZONE ONE
Casualty is Conscious.
Voluntary and Involuntary Muscle Control.

ZONE TWO
Casualty is Unconscious.
No Voluntary Muscle Control.

ZONE THREE
Casualty has stopped breathing.
Involuntary Muscle Control of Heart still Functioning.

ZONE FOUR
Casualty's Heart has Stopped Beating.

Fig.10. Conditional Zones of a Casualty

EMERGENCY DIAGNOSIS PROCEDURE

D Ensure there is no **Danger** to yourself or the casualty.

R Check for a **Response** from the casualty. Place your hands on the casualty's shoulders and gently shake them. At the same time loudly state a simple command such as "open your eyes" to determine if the casualty is conscious or unconscious (zone 1 or zone 2). If there is no response, shout for help in the local vicinity and proceed to Airway.

A If no response, clear and open the casualty's **Airway**.

When a person is unconscious, the voluntary muscles of the body relax, and the body will become generally limp and floppy. The tongue is a voluntary muscle and just like the arms and legs will relax. When the tongue relaxes it falls onto the back of the throat and causes an obstruction, thus closing the airway off.

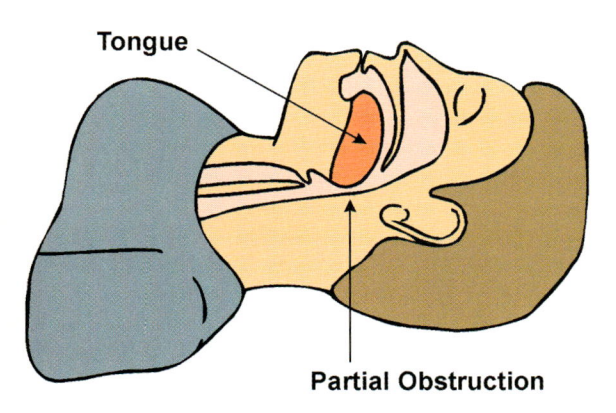

Fig.11. Closed Airway

As well as the tongue, there may also be foreign material or other obstructions inside the mouth such as dentures, broken teeth, chewing gum, saliva or vomit.

Obstruction of the airway due to the relaxed tongue is a major cause of death in the unconscious casualty and this problem must be dealt with immediately.

Opening the Airway

This is achieved by using the **head tilt - chin lift** procedure.

Inside the mouth, the tongue is connected to the jaw and if the chin is lifted upward, it will lift the tongue off the back of the throat. At the same time as the chin is lifted, the casualty's head should be tilted gently backward.

- Place the palm of one hand on the casualty's forehead, and gently tilt the casualty's head back. If there is an obvious visible obstruction inside the mouth, remove it. Lift the chin. If you suspect (due to the history of the accident) that the casualty may have head or neck injury, it is important that the movement is carried out slowly and carefully and only so far as to open the airway and not so far as to make any possible neck injury worse.

- Place two fingers of the other hand onto the bony prominence at the front of the casualty's chin. Do not press on the soft tissue under the chin as this will further obstruct the airway by pressing the tongue against the roof of the mouth.

Do not over extend or apply force to the neck when performing this technique. If you meet resistance to the head tilt, it usually indicates that the head is already well back. Continued tilting may cause further injury to the casualty.

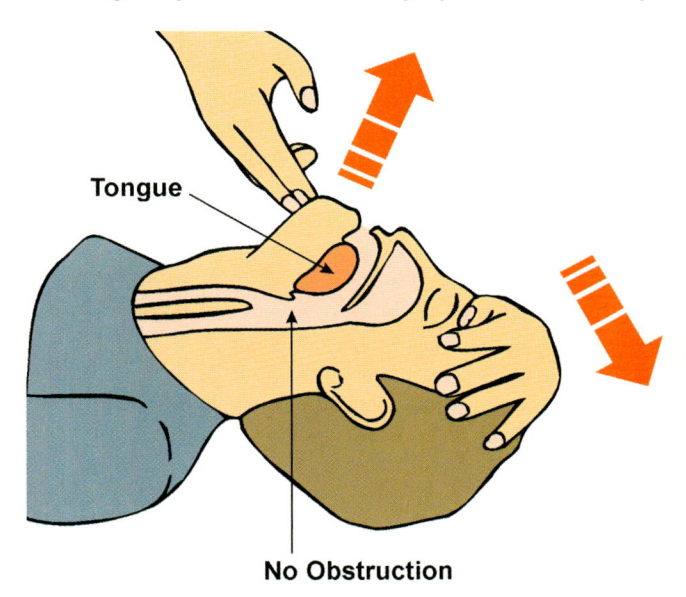

Fig.12. Opening the Airway

Removal of foreign objects from the mouth is best performed using the **finger sweep** technique.

- Insert your index finger into the casualty's mouth and sweep around the mouth in an attempt to hook the finger underneath the object and scoop it out.

Do not use your fingers to feel blindly around the back of the throat.

If an object is lodged firmly at the back of the throat, do not attempt to remove it with the finger sweep. Follow the procedures detailed for choking in an unconscious casualty (Page 4.2).

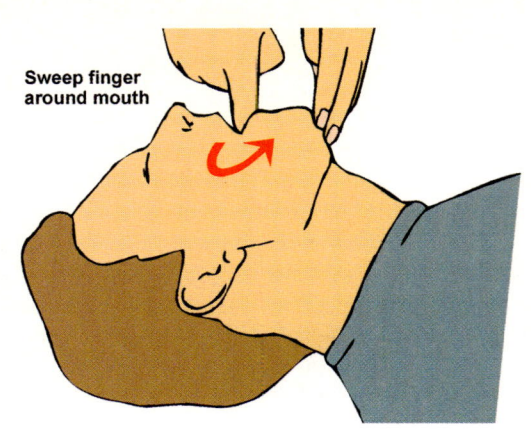

Fig. 13. Clearing an Obstruction

B Keeping the airway open, assess if the casualty is **Breathing** normally (more than the occasional gasp) by:

- Looking down the chest for any sign of movement.
- Listening for breathing sounds at the mouth.
- Feeling (with your cheek) for warm air being exhaled.

Look, listen and feel for no more than 10 seconds before deciding that normal breathing is absent.

If the casualty is breathing (more than an occasional gasp), treat as for the unconscious casualty (see section 9).

If the casualty is not breathing, send a bystander or helper for an ambulance and tell them to say that the casualty is not breathing. This specific information will help the ambulance service prioritise the call.

It is a fair assumption that by now, if the casualty is not breathing, the amount of oxygen in their blood will be down to a dangerously low level. It is therefore necessary at this stage to supply the casualty with oxygen by giving two effective breaths of artificial ventilation (see section 8).

C Assess if the casualty has **Circulation**. Look, listen and feel for normal breathing, coughing, movement, or any other signs of life. Assessment for circulation should take no more than 10 seconds.

If you are confident that the casualty has circulation, continue artificial ventilation and monitor the circulation every one minute.

If the casualty is not breathing and there are no signs of circulation (or you are at all unsure), chest compressions combined with artificial ventilation of the casualty's lungs will be necessary (see section 8).

When Do I Call for an Ambulance?

It is essential that professional help is called quickly if a casualty is not breathing. Therefore, if there is a bystander or helper at the scene, send them to call for an ambulance as soon as you know that the casualty is unresponsive and is not breathing.

If you are alone and the casualty is not breathing:

- If the likely cause of unconsciousness is:
  Alcohol or
  Drug intoxication;
  Drowning; or if it is an
  Infant or child; or
  Choking; or
  Trauma

  give artificial ventilation (see Appendix H•1 and section 8) and assess for signs of circulation (as above). Resuscitate the casualty with artificial ventilation and if appropriate with chest compressions for one minute, then leave the casualty to call for an ambulance. On return to the casualty, recheck A.B.C. and continue resuscitation as necessary (see section 8).

- If the likely cause of unconsciousness is not as above, the appointed person should assume that the casualty has a heart problem and go to call for an ambulance immediately it has been established that the casualty is not breathing. On return to the casualty, recheck A.B.C. and begin resuscitation as necessary (see section 8).

As HSE recommends that any appointed person working regularly alone has the means to summon help in an emergency, it is unlikely that an appointed person should need to leave any casualty.

Test Your Knowledge

1) If you are entirely alone with a non-breathing casualty, state the instances where you would give CPR for a minute before going to telephone for an ambulance:

a) ....   b) ....
c) ....   d) ....
e) ....   f) ....

The Unconscious Casualty

Unconsciousness can be a consequence of many injuries and sudden illnesses. The ability to deal promptly and effectively with an unconscious casualty is of great importance to all appointed persons

Unconsciousness is defined as an interruption in the normal activity of the brain. The brain is a very complex organ, in fact so complex that even today very little is known and understood about how it manages to perform so many intricate and precise tasks. The brain is responsible for the control and co-ordination of nearly all body functions and, like the master processing chip inside a computer, if it becomes damaged the whole system may crash.

Situated within the protective confines of the skull, the brain is further protected by layers of tissue called meninges which completely surround it and its connecting link with the body, the spinal cord. Further protection is provided by a layer of fluid which is situated between two layers of the meninges, called cerebro-spinal fluid, which acts as a shock absorber.

Although reasonably well-protected, the cells of the brain are so delicate they are still very vulnerable to damage, be it temporary or permanent.

Common Causes of Unconsciousness

There are many individual causes of unconsciousness, but in general there are three main reasons why the normal functioning of the brain could be interrupted: physical damage to brain tissue caused by a head injury or stroke; chemical damage to brain tissue caused by increased levels of toxin or chemical substances in the blood stream; and lack of oxygen to brain tissue caused by asphyxiation or blood loss.

There are ten main common causes of unconsciousness. **F**ainting, **I**nfections, **S**troke, **H**ead injury, **S**hock, **H**eart attack, **A**sphyxia, **P**oisoning, **E**pilepsy and **D**iabetes. (F.I.S.H. S.H.A.P.E.D)

1. Fainting

This usually occurs when the oxygen supply to the brain is reduced. There are many things which could stimulate this such as lack of physical activity, and a warm, stuffy environment, but perhaps the commonest cause is emotional distress.

Most people have experienced some degree of overwhelming emotional distress in their lives, such as news of a bereavement, a good telling off by the boss at work or just reading their recent council tax bill. When subject to overwhelming emotional distress the body has a particular way of dealing with it. It is an involuntary or automatic response called the 'fight or flight syndrome' where the body quickly releases large amounts of chemical substances (one of which is called adrenalin) into the body tissues. These chemical substances, along with nervous impulses, cause a wide variety of physical reactions to occur inside the body, such as an increase in the blood pressure, an increase in heart and breathing rates, a reduction in blood flow to the skin and guts and the stimulation of the sweating mechanism.

If a person is in an upright posture when this occurs, the forces of gravity prevent much of the blood returning up to the heart and head. This brief lack of blood and oxygen to the brain causes dizziness and eventually interrupts brain activity so much that unconsciousness can result.

This mild form of unconsciousness associated with a simple faint is usually brief and treatment involves returning blood flow and oxygen supply to the brain.

- Lay the casualty down on their back.
- Keep the airway open and clear and loosen any tight or restrictive clothing.
- Elevate their legs to improve the return of blood to the top half of the body.

If recovery is swift, no further treatment is usually required. If the faint or dizzy spell is persistent or occurs on a frequent basis, the casualty should be advised to see a doctor at the earliest possible opportunity. If the unconsciousness lasts for more than just a few minutes, place the casualty in the recovery position and call for an ambulance.

2. Infections

When the body is invaded by microscopic organisms such as viruses and bacteria, it reacts in many different ways to fight off the infection, such as the production of antibodies and the raising of body temperature. If the infection is severe and spreads to the brain tissue, unconsciousness can result.

3. Stroke

Otherwise known as a cerebro-vascular accident (CVA), a stroke occurs when small blood vessels in the brain become obstructed (usually due to a blood clot). This obstruction will cause a reduction or absolute stoppage of blood supply to the brain tissue, resulting in oxygen deprivation and tissue death. Furthermore, pressure builds up behind the blockage in the blood vessel which causes it to distend and eventually rupture. The effects of a stroke depend primarily on how much, and which part, of the brain is affected, but in many cases it will interfere with the normal activity of the brain and result in unconsciousness.

4. Head Injuries

One of the most common causes of unconsciousness, but in many cases it is only temporary and reversible. The duration and depth of the resulting unconsciousness depends on the severity of the subsequent brain damage.

5. Shock

There are many different types of shock. The body's reaction to overwhelming emotional circumstances is known as emotional or neurogenic shock (as described in fainting above). True or hypovolaemic shock develops when the body loses circulating fluid, such as blood. This would reduce blood pressure and oxygen supply to vital areas, thus causing an interference in the normal activity of the brain and unconsciousness.

6. Heart Attack

This occurs when the heart muscle is starved of oxygen, usually due to a blockage in the arteries (coronary) which supply it with blood. If the muscle cells in the heart are starved of oxygen they will not function correctly and therefore the heart beat becomes weak and irregular. This lowers blood pressure and reduces blood flow to the brain.

7. Asphyxia

If the blood is unable to obtain sufficient oxygen for whatever reason, it will follow that there will be a reduction on the oxygen supply to the brain, eventually resulting in unconsciousness.

8. Poisoning

When harmful substances enter the body they can easily work themselves into the blood stream which is a direct and unobstructed route to the vital organs, especially the brain.

9. Epilepsy

Epilepsy is described as a tendency to experience repeated muscular contractions or convulsions which are due to an internal problem in the brain. There are many different types of epilepsy, each with its own particular traits and recognition points, but all types involve some degree of electrical disturbance in the brain, many of which cause some degree of unconsciousness.

10. Diabetes

This is a condition in which the body fails to regulate the amount of sugar (glucose) in the blood stream. If the blood sugar level rises or falls outside of certain parameters it can have a severe and adverse effect on the body, in particular brain activity.

Treatment of Unconsciousness

In most cases of unconsciousness, there is very little an appointed person can do to reverse the primary cause, therefore general treatment revolves around the main problem associated with the unconsciousness itself - airway obstruction.

After performing the emergency diagnosis (unresponsive but breathing and pulse present):

1. Perform a Top-to-Toe Examination

This is a systematic and methodical assessment of the casualty's body to determine the presence or absence of injuries, and evidence of other important details relating to the casualty.

It is logical that in any examination of a casualty the most serious and life threatening injuries are found first. When carrying out the examination, the appointed person should always bear in mind the cause and history of the accident which will have great significance on exactly where and what type of injuries the casualty may have sustained. For example, a casualty who has been subject to direct impact and violence to the body is much more likely to have sustained broken bones than a casualty who has collapsed due to overheating. A casualty who was subject to blast and fragmentation is much more likely to sustain open wounds than a casualty who has suffered an allergic reaction to an insect sting, and so on.

The examination will involve the use of the

appointed person's senses of touch, sight and smell and it is carried out in two stages.

Use both hands together to compare one side of the body to the other. Feel underneath clothing if necessary. Use the tips of your fingers where possible to increase sensitivity.

If necessary, remove or re-position any clothing which obstructs clear vision of the skin and body surface in areas where you suspect an injury to be present.

If available, it may be beneficial to put on a pair of protective examination gloves before commencing a top-to-toe examination of a casualty.

Stage 1

Check quickly but thoroughly all the way down the body (including the limbs) for any sign of serious bleeding. If serious bleeding is found, deal with it immediately.

Stage 2

Check the body again from the head to the feet for other injuries and any evidence relating to the possible cause of the unconsciousness.

- Head & Neck

    Feel for any deformity, swelling, lumps, and indentations.

    Look for any minor bleeding, bruising or deformities. Look for any liquid or blood leaking from the eyes, ears or nose.

    Look at the eyes to see if they are bloodshot.

    Look for a Medic-Alert or other talisman around the casualty's neck. This could give information on any medical condition which the casualty suffers from, such as epilepsy, diabetes or allergies.

    Smell the casualty's breath for alcohol or unusual smells such as acetone (like nail varnish remover).

- Shoulders

    Feel for any deformity and swelling, especially around the collar bones.

    Look for any minor bleeding and bruising.

- Chest

    Feel for any deformities.

    Look for any unnatural movement of the chest wall and for any minor bleeding.

- Abdomen

    Feel for any deformity or hard areas (which could indicate internal injury) and for any minor bleeding.

- Hips

    Feel for any deformity.

    Look for any minor bleeding.

    Look for any damp patches in the groin area which may indicate that the casualty has urinated.

    Remove any bulky or sharp objects from the casualty's pockets which may cause injury when rolling into the recovery position. Ensure that any objects which are removed are kept safe and passed on to the ambulance service when they arrive. If possible, put the objects into a container or envelope, label it with the casualty's details and have a second person witness that your actions were necessary and above-board.

- Arms & Hands

    Feel for any deformity or swelling.

    Look for any minor bleeding and for a Medic-Alert or other talisman around the wrist.

- Legs & Feet

    Feel for any deformity or swelling.

    Look for any minor bleeding, or dampness between the legs.

Exactly how long this check should take and how thorough it should be again depends primarily on the history. If a casualty has been subject to blast and fragmentation, the damage to the body could be extensive and therefore more time should be taken. If a casualty has only fainted, damage to the body would be minimal therefore less time would be taken. If the examination is lengthy, keep going back to check the airway and breathing every minute or so. It would be poor technique to spend ten minutes performing a thorough examination only to find out that the casualty stopped breathing eight minutes ago.

If any serious injuries are found during the examination, it may be necessary to treat them before further treatment for the unconsciousness continues. If this is so, keep a close watch on the airway and breathing throughout treatment.

Warning key rings, bracelets and necklaces such as Medic-Alert and S.O.S. talisman provide details of medical information pertaining to the person carrying or wearing it. Commonest indications they give are for diabetes, epilepsy and allergies.

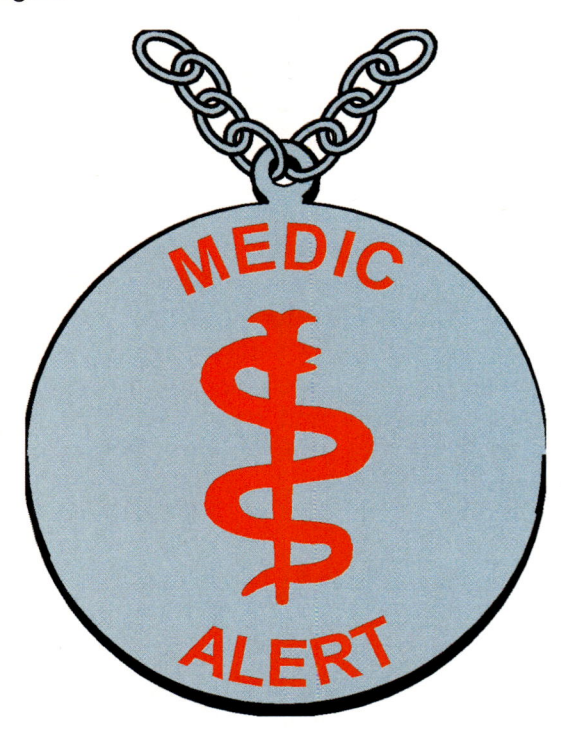

Fig.14. Medic-Alert

2. Place the Casualty in the Recovery Position

Without specialised equipment it can be very dangerous to leave an unconscious casualty laid on their back.

- Even with the airway extended, the tongue could still slightly close off the airway.
- If the casualty should suddenly vomit, it would cause airway obstruction and the vomit may be inhaled.
- Saliva which secretes into the mouth would drain to the back of the throat and be inhaled.

Bearing these factors in mind, unconscious casualties should be placed in a position which alleviates these potential problems - the Recovery Position.

There are many different variations of the recovery position, each with their own individual attributes and benefits. Regardless of which individual position is used, there are six specific criteria which should be observed.

- The position is as near true lateral position as possible with the head dependent to allow free drainage of fluid.
- The position should be stable.
- Any pressure on the chest which impairs breathing should be avoided.
- It should be possible to turn the casualty onto the side and return to the back easily and safely having particular regard to the possibility of a neck or spine injury.
- Good observation and access to the airway should be possible.
- The position itself should not give rise to any injury to the casualty.

To turn a casualty into the recovery position:

- Kneel next to the casualty and raise the arm which is nearest to you, out to the side. This ensures that the casualty will not roll on to the arm which could restrict breathing.

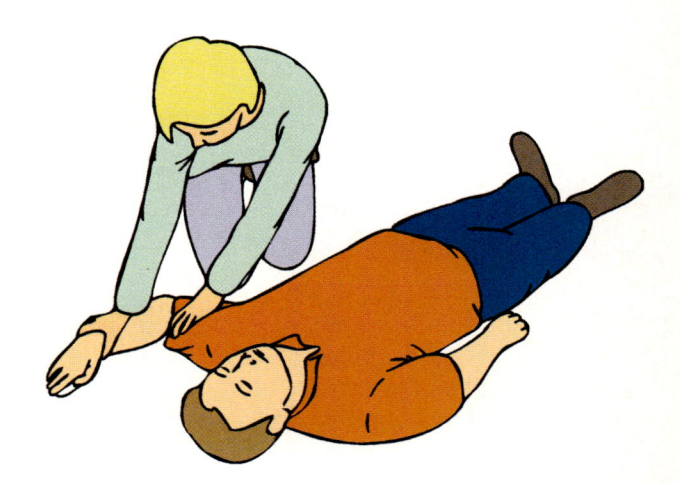

- Reach across the casualty, lift up their hand (palm-to-palm) and gently place the back of their hand against the side of their face. If the casualty is wearing a ring which could scratch their face, carefully turn it around so the sharp or bulky part is facing the palm.

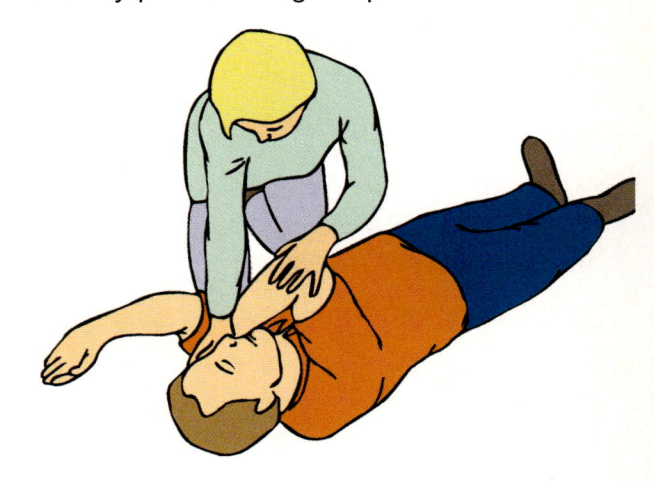

- Keeping this hand in position to support the head, lift the opposite knee with the other hand. The bent leg will now provide a lever with which to roll the casualty.

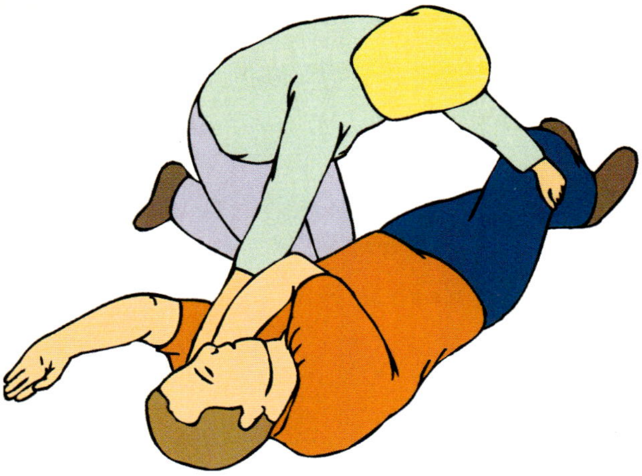

Fig.15. Turning a casualty into the Recovery Position

- Supporting the head with one hand, gently pull the knee towards you and the casualty will begin to turn. Allow the casualty to turn approximately three quarters of the way over onto their front. By now the knee on which you were pulling should be in contact with the floor.

- Gently remove your hand from underneath the cheek and allow the casualty's head to rest on the back of their hand. Gently tilt the head back to ensure the airway remains open and re-check breathing.

- Pull up on the knee of the upper leg so the hip and knee are bent at approximately right angles. This bent leg will stop the casualty rolling over completely onto their front.

- Check the circulation in the arm which passes under the casualty's body by feeling for the radial pulse at the wrist. If the pulse is absent or there is any sign that circulation into the arm is interrupted, slightly reposition the arm until normal circulation returns.

- If the casualty has to be kept in the recovery position for more than 30 minutes, if injuries permit they should be turned onto the opposite side - this relieves pressure on the circulation of the lower arm.

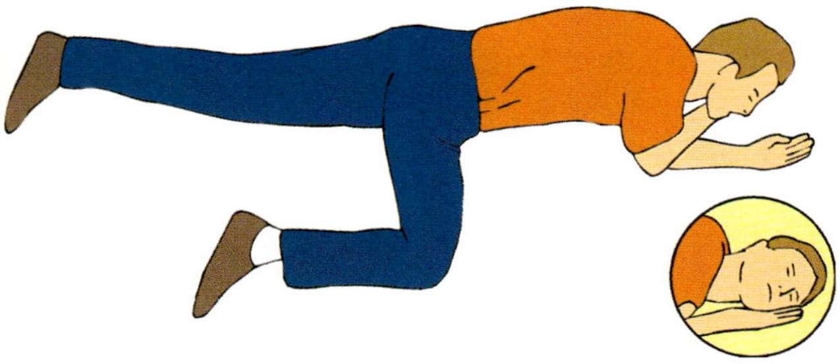

Fig.16. The Recovery Position

Modifying the Recovery Position

In some cases the unconscious casualty may already be lying on their front when you arrive on the scene. If this is so,

- Carry out the A.B.C. of emergency diagnosis. If the casualty is not breathing, they must be carefully turned onto their back for resuscitation.

If the casualty is breathing, it is unnecessary to turn them on to their back, just to turn them back on to their front. A modified recovery position can be achieved by simply and gently repositioning their limbs.

- Note which way the head is already turned and carefully move the hand on this side between the face and the ground. Ensure that the airway remains open.

- Bend and raise the knee on the same side. This will lift the casualty's abdomen and lower chest off the ground and allow for unrestricted breathing.

- Ensure the arm on the opposite side of the body is in a safe position and check the radial pulse to ensure that circulation is not impeded.

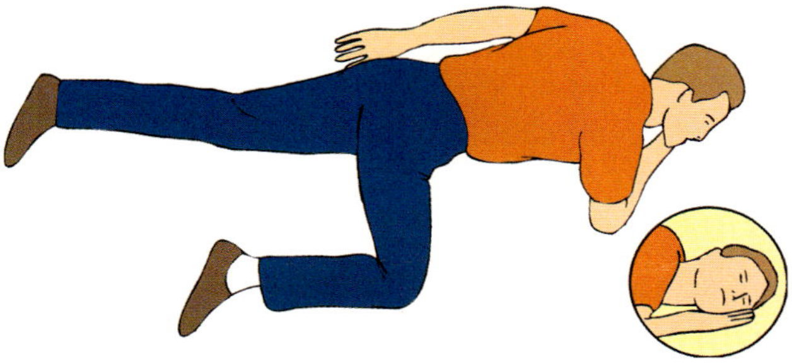

Fig.17. Modified Recovery Position

In some cases, the top-to-toe examination of the casualty may have discovered the presence of other injuries, in particular broken bones (fractures).

If you suspect fractures to the arms or legs, the position may again need to be modified to take account of the injury. Remember, nothing takes priority over the casualty's airway and breathing, but when modifying the position, try to move the injured area as little as possible.

The Spinal Injury Recovery Position

Perhaps the most daunting situation with an unconscious casualty is when spinal injuries are suspected. In many cases it may be impossible for the appointed person to tell if the casualty's back or neck is injured. If the history and circumstances of the accident indicate that the casualty has been subject to violence or direct impact (such as a fall or being hit by a falling object), the golden rule is to always suspect that the spine may be damaged and to take this into account when rolling the casualty over.

The turning process for the recovery position described above (using the knee as a lever) causes the spine to twist and this is likely to make a back injury worse. If there are helpers around, however, the turning process can be achieved without twisting or bending the back at all. A minimum of three people are required to perform this technique safely.

To turn an unconscious casualty into this position:

- With the casualty laid on their back, very gently straighten the limbs in line with the body.

- One person (the team leader) should kneel at the head of the casualty, facing down the mid line of the casualty's body, holding the casualty's head in a neutral, mid-line position. The hands should be placed over the casualty's ears to ensure a firm but gentle grip.

- A second person should kneel beside the casualty (in line with the chest) and move the nearest arm out to the side. They should then lean over the casualty and gently slide their hands under the casualty's far shoulder and hip.

- A third person should kneel at the same side of the casualty (in line with the legs) and lean over the casualty, sliding their hands gently under the casualty's far hip and lower leg.

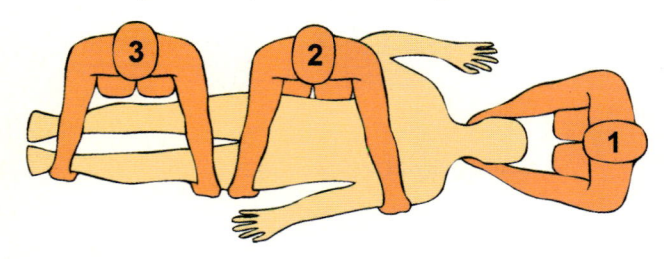

Fig.18. Positions for turning - Spinal Injury Recovery Position

- Person number 1 should call out the timing for the turn, e.g. ready... steady... turn. This will ensure that persons 2 and 3 start pulling at the same time.

- Persons 2 and 3 should now pull the casualty toward themselves, ensuring that they are pulling at the same speed to ensure the whole body remains straight. Person number 1 should ensure that as the body is turned, the nose remains constantly on the mid line of the body, thus not allowing the neck to twist or bend.

The turning process should be slow enough to ensure the whole body is 'log rolled' 90 degrees until the casualty is laid on their side.

- Once over on their side, padding should be inserted between the ground and the casualty's lower cheek to ensure that the head does not fall, twisting the neck.

The airway should be assessed and a check made to ensure there is no restriction on movement of the chest wall.

Circulation in the lower arm should be checked for impediment by feeling the radial pulse.

- Padding should now be placed around the casualty to stabilise the position.

3. Perform a Head to Heel Examination

Now that the casualty has been turned over, a further examination for injuries should be carried out down the casualty's back.

The examination should look for open wounds, bleeding, swelling, deformity and discolouration of the skin. If clothing impedes visual inspection, it should be carefully adjusted or removed if necessary. If any injuries are found, treat accordingly.

4. Carry out Basic Observations

The casualty must now be monitored regularly for any sign of change in their condition. A written record should be made of the findings and passed on to the ambulance service when they arrive.

- **Information to Record**

  - A brief history of the accident, and if possible the personal details of the casualty such as name, address, age, etc.
  - The nature and approximate time of the accident.
  - Notes about any injuries found on the casualty, or any evidence which helps determine the cause of unconsciousness. Details of any medication which the casualty takes or allergies they have (if known).
  - Details of any treatment given.

- **Observations to Record**

There are five basic observations to record. Breathing, pulse, pupils, pallor and response.

  - Breathing. Note details of its rate, depth and regularity. Remember, the normal breathing rate for an adult at rest is 14 to 18 breaths per minute.

  - Pulse. Note details of its rate (speed), strength and regularity. Remember, the normal pulse rate for an adult at rest is 60 to 80 beats per minute.

  - Pupils. Note if they are equal in size and if they react to light. Irregular or fixed pupils often indicate that the brain is damaged in some way.

  - Pallor. Note the colour of the casualty's skin.

Is it pale, flushed, or normal? Look for blueness, especially at the extremities (cyanosis). Feel the temperature of the casualty's face. Is it warm, cold or normal?

- Level of response. This helps determine the depth of unconsciousness.

    A - Are they alert and opening their eyes spontaneously?

    V - Do they respond to your voice? Give them simple commands such as "open your eyes".

    P - Do they respond to painful stimuli? Gently pinch the very end of the casualty's ear lobe. Look for an automatic reflex such as a flinch of the eye, movement of the facial muscles or perhaps even a groan.

    U - Are they unresponsive to all stimuli?

You must only leave an unconscious casualty if it is absolutely necessary, e.g. when you are alone and have to go and call for an ambulance. If you must leave the casualty, ensure that they are in the recovery position before you leave. It may be necessary to place support behind the casualty to make the position more stable and ensure that they cannot roll over onto their back in your absence.

If at any time the casualty should stop breathing, gently but quickly roll them back onto their back and commence resuscitation as appropriate.

Examining a casualty

Is summed up as a **primary survey**, as per the flowchart of page 3.4, which follows the current Resuscitation Council protocols, then a **secondary survey**.

1. Listen to the history of the accident and look for external clues.
2. If an accident, find out how it happened and the forces involved.
3. Look for signs and symptoms.
4. Examine the casualty.

Test Your Knowledge

1) You are dealing with a casualty who is breathing but unconscious. There are no obvious injuries. You should now (please tick one answer):

    a) Go and phone for an ambulance.
    b) Fill out the accident report book.
    c) Place the casualty into the recovery position.
    d) Avoid moving them in case you make the condition worse.

2) From the list below, tick the four aspects that you consider to be the most important when dealing with an unconscious casualty:

    a) Keep the casualty warm
    b) Complete the accident book
    c) Place in the recovery position
    d) Phone for an ambulance
    e) Resuscitate if necessary
    f) Establish levels of responsiveness
    g) Carry out general body check/observations
    h) Maintain airway

3) You are dealing with a casualty who is breathing but unconscious.

    a) What position should you place the casualty in? ....
    b) Give two reasons why this position should be used.

        i ....
        ii ....

4) When dealing with an unconscious casualty, there are four levels of responsiveness. What are they?

    A ....V ....P ....U ....

Wounds and Bleeding

Bleeding is a very common type of injury and most appointed persons in the workplace will at some point have to deal with an open wound.

Whenever blood vessels are punctured, split, torn, cut or severed, the blood inside will leak out. Exactly how much blood is lost from a wound depends largely on the type and size of blood vessels which have been damaged.

Types of Bleeding

1. Arterial Bleeding

The blood inside arteries is usually under a high degree of pressure so when an artery is damaged the resulting blood loss can be very serious. This type of bleeding can be very difficult to control, especially if large arteries are damaged.

> In some cases of severe external bleeding, it is possible to see the blood from a damaged artery spurting from the wound in time with the heart beat. The majority of arteries in the body carry oxygenated blood which usually gives arterial bleeding a very bright red appearance.

2. Venous Bleeding

The blood inside veins is not usually under a high degree of pressure so when a vein is damaged the resulting blood loss is not as serious as that from a similar-sized artery. As the pressure is low, this type of bleeding is fairly easy to control. Again, due to the lower pressure, the blood from a vein will flow rather than spurt from the wound. The majority of veins carry de-oxygenated blood which usually gives a dark red appearance.

3. Capillary Bleeding

Bleeding from capillaries is not usually serious and control can be achieved with simple techniques.

In general, the higher the degree of blood pressure inside the blood vessel, the quicker the blood loss will be.

Minor Wounds

Minor wounds such as small cuts, scratches and grazes are common injuries but treatment is simple.

- Gently clean the wound with fresh tap water or, if water is not available, use an individually wrapped moist cleansing wipe from the first aid kit. When clean, dry the area with the gauze pad of a sterile dressing.

- Apply a suitably-sized adhesive dressing over the wound, ensuring that all the wound is covered and the adhesive element of the dressing does not come into contact with the wound itself.

- If a suitable adhesive dressing is not available, use a sterile wound dressing. The bleeding will usually stop quickly due to the natural clotting reaction of the blood

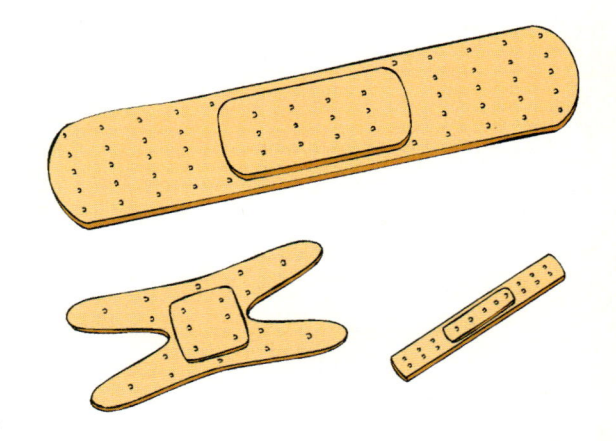

- Advise the casualty to watch out for signs of infection in the wound such as tenderness, swelling, reddening or pus oozing from the wound. Advise the casualty to see their doctor if infection becomes evident. In some cases, the casualty may need to have a tetanus injection following even the most minor wound. If there is a risk from tetanus and the casualty does not know if they are up to date with their immunisation, the casualty should again be advised to seek further medical aid from their doctor.

Advise the casualty to return to you if bleeding persists.

- Record the details in the accident book.

Major Wounds

There is no specific dividing line between what constitutes a minor wound and what constitutes a major wound, but in the context of most first aid treatments major wounds are generally classified as those which require more than just the application of a simple adhesive dressing, i.e. bleeding from arteries and veins.

There are three main elements to the treatment of major wounds. **R**est, **E**levation and **D**irect Pressure (R.E.D.)

1. Rest the Casualty

As already explained, the speed of blood loss from a wound will be directly proportional to the pressure of blood inside the damaged blood vessels, therefore factors which raise the blood pressure unnecessarily should be avoided. These include emotional distress and physical activity.

To overcome these factors, the casualty should be:

- allowed to adopt a comfortable resting position usually sitting down, although in cases where shock develops, laying down with the legs slightly elevated;
- reassured as to the severity of the injury and the competence of the appointed person.

2. Elevate the Wound

If the wound is supported at a level above that of the heart, blood will have to travel upwards to reach the wound. The increased gravitational effect will help reduce the blood flow (and pressure) to the wound. If elevation of the wound is not possible due to the nature or location of the wound, try at least to get the wound level with the heart and not below it.

If there is a suspected broken bone in the area of the wound (open fracture), ensure that the bone is completely immobilised before elevation otherwise movement of the bone ends will cause more damage to the surrounding tissue and make the bleeding worse. If in doubt, do not elevate open fractures.

3. Apply Direct Pressure

This is the main principle in the control of bleeding. The application of counter pressure on the wound will reduce the pressure and speed at which blood exits, just like putting your thumb over the end of a hose pipe.

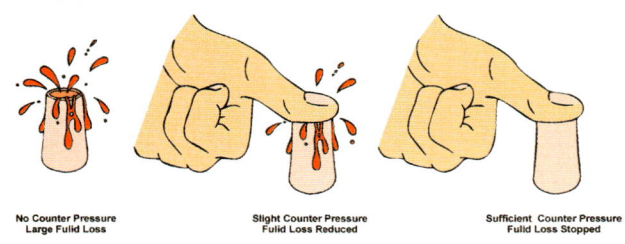

Fig.19. The Principle of Counter Pressure

Exactly how much counter pressure is required will be entirely dependent on the pressure at which the blood comes out of the damaged blood vessels. Arterial bleeding often requires a high degree of counter pressure to stop the blood flow.

Before applying a pressure dressing, examine the wound for any embedded objects. If an object is embedded in the wound e.g. metal or glass, an alternative method of application will be necessary (see Embedded Objects).

Pressure should be applied to an open wound using a sterile wound dressing. Wound dressings come in a huge variety of shapes and sizes and most first aid kits contain a good selection. The Health and Safety Executive issue guidance to employers which recommends that two approximate sizes of wound dressing should be made available, 12cm x 12cm and 18cm x 18cm. Further to this, wound dressings should be sterile, individually wrapped and unmedicated.

The chosen dressing should, if possible, be large enough to cover the entire wound. If the wound is very large, it may take multiple dressings to ensure complete coverage.

There are many different methods of applying wound dressings, but regardless of which method is used, the following principles must apply:

- carefully remove or cut away all clothing around the wound. A dressing should not be used over the top of clothing as this may reduce its effect;
- sterility of the dressing should be maintained. Try not to touch the face of the sterile pad when unwrapping and applying the dressing;
- the pad of the dressing should be placed in a central position over the wound and all the wound should be covered;
- the tails should be wrapped around without twisting or screwing up. This will ensure that the tails do not dig in and, in the case of a limb, will reduce the chances of circulation impediment;
- when applied, the tails should cover all the pad and the pressure should be evenly distributed across all the pad. If pressure is only applied in the middle, blood will seep out from the sides;
- the tail ends should be secured in position to prevent them from unwrapping. This is usually achieved by tying a knot or using a safety pin from the first aid kit;

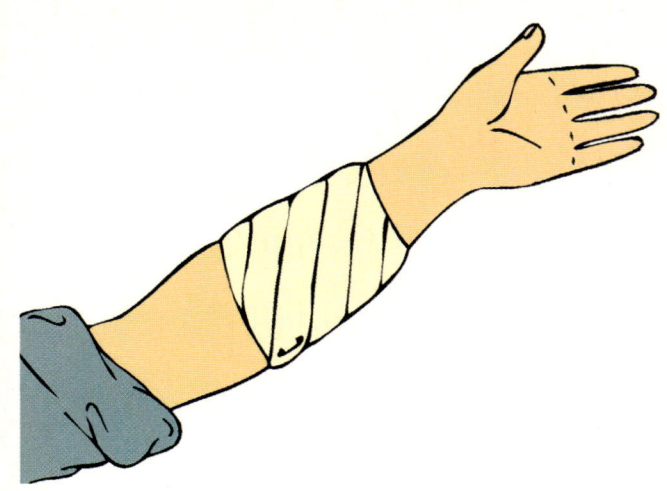

Fig.20. Pressure Dressing

- in cases of bandages to the limbs, check the circulation in the limb once the bandage is applied. If the bandage is too tight it could cut off the circulation, making the limb go pale and cold. The casualty may also begin to sense a numbness or tingling sensation in the limb. If circulation is impeded, the dressing may have to be loosened slightly;
- monitor the dressing to ensure that the bleeding is controlled;
- if one dressing is insufficient to control the bleeding, blood will eventually seep through.

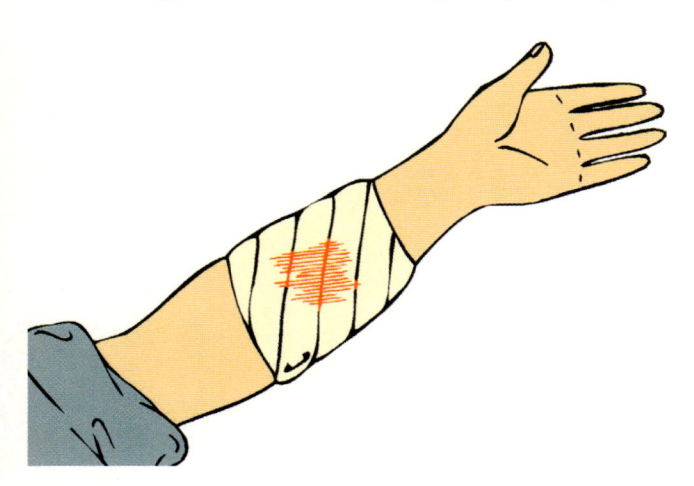

If this occurs, apply a second dressing over the top of the first, in exactly the same way. Do not remove the initial dressing. The combined pressure from two pressure bandages may be enough to stop the bleeding;

- if blood seeps through the second dressing, apply a third dressing over the top of the second. Do not remove the second dressing. The combined pressure from three bandages may be enough to stop the bleeding;
- if the bleeding is so severe that it begins to seep through a second pressure bandage, or at any time the casualty begins to show signs of shock, call for an ambulance.

Soggy dressings after treating bleeding

The first aider should, if blood seeps through two dressings, remove them and apply a new one. (If the original dressing was applied accurately to the point of bleeding with appropriate pressure – firm enough to stop bleeding but not so firm as to cut off circulation – this should not be necessary.)

Indirect Pressure (Pressure Points)

In extreme cases, blood may seep through the third pressure bandage. A fourth dressing over the top of the third is unlikely to add any more significant pressure, therefore the only course of action remaining is to reduce the blood flow to the wound.

Arteries carry blood to all parts of the body. The principle of indirect pressure is to apply pressure not to the wound, but to the artery which supplies the wound with blood. Indirect pressure to control bleeding is applied on an artery at a point where it passes over a bone - a 'pressure point'.

Blood flow is reduced at point of pressure

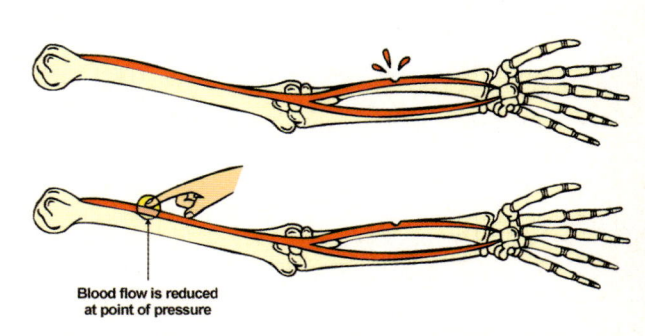

Fig.21. The Principle of Indirect Pressure (Pressure Points)

Pressure points can be found all over the body but first aid is generally limited to the use of two. The brachial pressure point in the upper arm and the femoral pressure point in the groin.

1. The Brachial Pressure Point

The brachial pressure point can be located on the brachial artery in the upper arm. The brachial artery lies between the upper arm muscle (biceps) and the upper arm bone (humerus). If pressure is applied in the correct place, the appointed person should be able to feel the brachial pulse.

Pressure is applied by gripping around the upper arm, with the finger tips pressing directly on the artery. In most cases it is necessary to remove any clothing from the upper arm. Applying pressure over clothing can make the technique very difficult.

2. The Femoral Pressure Point

The femoral pressure point can be located on the femoral artery in the upper leg. The femoral artery runs from the front of the groin, down the inner aspect of the upper leg and ends at the back of the knee. The artery comes closest to the surface of the body at the front of the groin. If pressure is applied in the correct place, the appointed person should be able to feel the femoral pulse.

Pressure is applied by gripping around the top of the leg, with the thumbs pressing down on the artery. In most cases it is necessary to work underneath clothing in the groin region. Applying pressure over clothing can make the technique very difficult.

Do not apply pressure with the heel of a boot or other hard object such as a piece of wood as this can cause severe damage to the blood vessels and nerves.

Firm, steady pressure should be applied to a pressure point for 10 to 15 minutes. This will allow time for the clotting process to work at the site of the wound. Release of pressure should be slow, thus allowing the blood to gently flow back to the wound and minimising any disturbance of the clotting. If fresh blood begins to seep back through the third dressing, re-apply the pressure for a further 10 to 15 minutes.

Embedded Objects

In some cases there may be an embedded object in a wound, such as metal or glass. **Under no circumstances should the appointed person attempt to remove the embedded object** as this can often make the problem worse by causing more damage and increasing the bleeding.

The method of application of pressure to a wound with an embedded object must be modified in such a way that the dressing does not push the object further in, yet still applies sufficient pressure to reduce or stop the bleeding.

- Place a rolled-up sterile dressing at one side of the wound. Ensure that it is placed close up to the embedded object at the edge of the wound.
- Place a second rolled-up dressing at the opposite side of the wound, again close up to the embedded object. The two rolled-up bandages should be higher than the embedded object, thus ensuring clearance for the last stage.

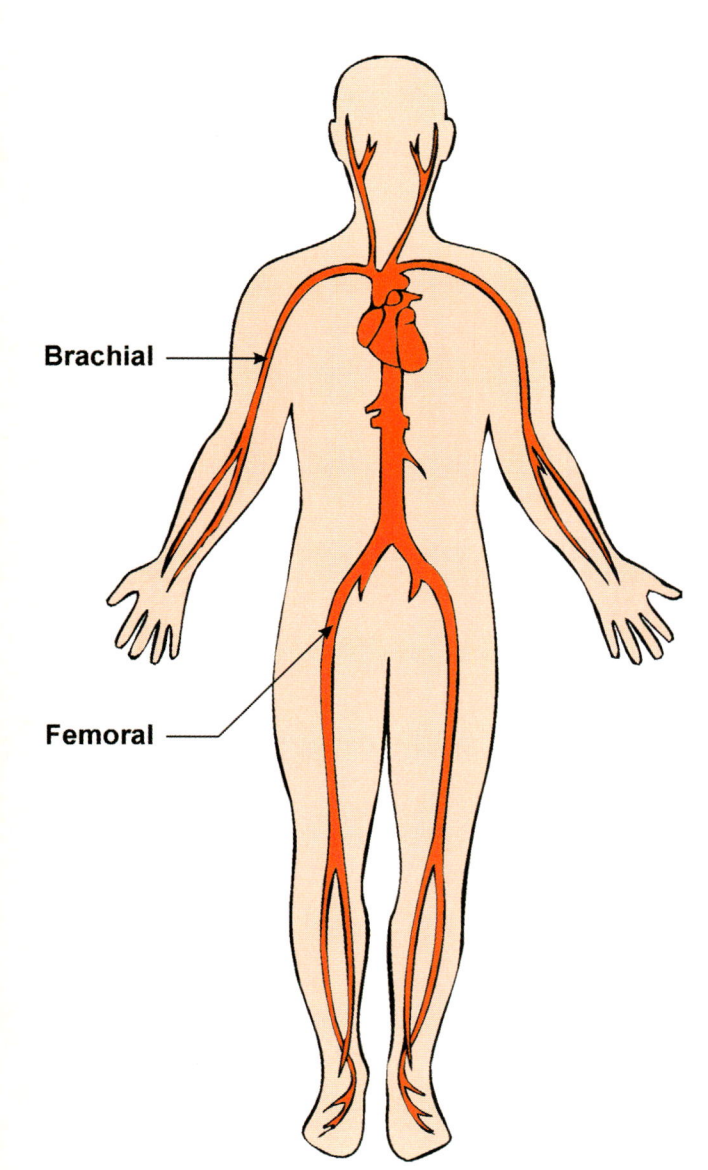

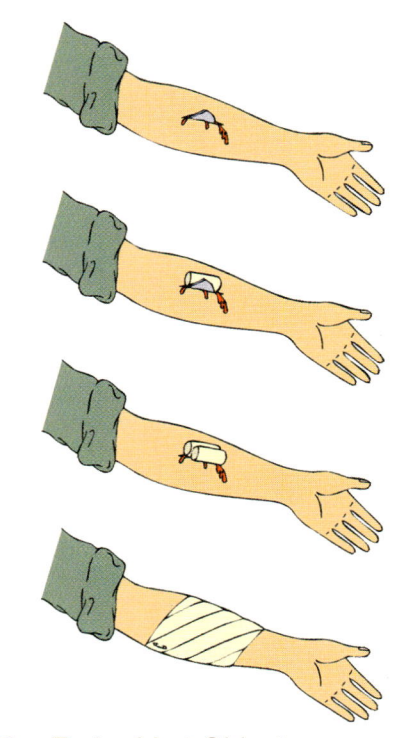

Fig.22. Pressure Points

Fig.23. The Embedded Object

- Place a wound dressing over the top and secure in place. When applying pressure, do not allow the top dressing to press directly onto the embedded object.
- If the object protrudes more than a couple of inches and rises above the level of the rolled-up dressings, do not cover the protruding part. Simply secure the top dressing in place, working around the object.

If an object should perforate completely through a limb, the treatment for the embedded object should be carried out at both the entry and exit points.

If the bandaging technique around a foreign or perforating object is done correctly, not only will it control the bleeding but it will also stabilise the object and stop it from moving around, preventing further damage.

Control of Bleeding from Limbs

- Put the casualty at rest. Sit or lay them down and reassure them.
- Elevate the wound above the level of the heart if possible.
- Examine the wound for any embedded object.
- Apply direct pressure to the wound with a wound dressing.
- If the wound is to an arm and the bleeding is controlled, support the arm in an elevation sling.
- If blood seeps through the first dressing, apply a second on top of the first.
- If blood seeps through the second dressing apply a third on top of the second.
- If blood seeps through the third dressing, use indirect pressure on the nearest pressure point.

Bleeding from the Palm

The palm of the hand can be a particularly tricky part of the body to bandage, therefore a slightly different method of applying direct pressure may be needed.

If the wound is across the palm:

- Press a sterile dressing over the wound and ask the casualty to clench their fist around it. This will ensure that the wound does not gape open.
- Bandage firmly around the whole fist to maintain the pressure on the dressing.
- If the casualty is unable to clench their fist (perhaps due to broken bones to the hand or fingers), ask the casualty to hold the dressing in place and apply pressure with their uninjured hand.
- In many cases of wounds to the hand and fingers, elevation can be maintained in an elevation sling.

If the wound is down the palm:

- Place a sterile dressing over the wound and simply bandage in place around the hand, keeping the fingers straight. If the fist is allowed to clench, it may make the wound gape open.
- Apply an elevation sling.

Amputations

If a part of the body has been amputated, treat the wound with rest, elevation, direct pressure and if necessary indirect pressure on the appropriate pressure point.

No matter how bad things may look, it is often possible for amputated parts to be re-attached, especially if they have been looked after in the correct way.

- It is important that the part is kept dry, **so do not wash it**. It should be wrapped in polythene or placed in a thin waterproof bag.
- It is also important that the part be kept cold (but not frozen), so secondly the part should be wrapped in a piece of cloth then placed in another container and surrounded by crushed ice if available.
- Mark the container containing the amputated part with the name of the casualty and the time of amputation (if known) and ensure that it is passed on to the ambulance service when they arrive.

Impalement

If a casualty is impaled on an object, do not attempt to separate them from the object as this is likely to make the injury and bleeding much worse.

- Make the casualty as comfortable as possible and, if necessary, support their body weight to relieve any tearing of the impaled part.
- Try to control any bleeding with wound dressings and, if necessary, pressure points.
- When calling for an ambulance, ensure that full details are passed on about the accident as specialist cutting tools may be needed to free the casualty.

Bleeding from the Scalp

The scalp has a very good blood supply and all wounds to the head can bleed profusely. In many cases, scalp wounds look a lot worse than they actually are but it must be remembered that with any head injury there may be some degree of damage to the brain such as concussion (see section 9).

- Make the casualty comfortable and reassure them.
- Apply a sterile dressing over the wound and bandage securely in place, applying sufficient pressure to stop the bleeding.
- Monitor the casualty for other signs and symptoms of head injury (see section 9) and treat accordingly.
- If the bleeding is controlled and there are no signs of concussion, take the casualty to hospital for further assessment and treatment.
- If the casualty becomes unconscious, place them into the recovery position and call for an ambulance.

Bleeding from the Nose

Nose bleeds are most commonly associated with blows to the head and face although some people are prone to spontaneous nose bleeds due to no apparent reason. Blood loss occurs from very small blood vessels inside the nasal cavity.

- Sit the casualty down and lean them forward. Encourage them to spit out any blood which may be in the mouth, not to swallow it. Give the casualty a receptacle or dressing to spit the blood into.
- Advise the casualty to breathe through their mouth and pinch together the soft part of the nostrils and keep them sealed off for 10 to 15 minutes to allow time for the blood to clot.

Do not attempt to plug the nostrils.

- After 10 to 15 minutes, release the nostrils and if bleeding persists, repeat the pinching process. If bleeding still persists, take the casualty to hospital for further assessment and treatment.
- If the nose bleed was caused by direct violence, monitor the casualty for any other signs of head injury (see section 9) and treat accordingly.
- If the bleeding stops, get the casualty to clean blood from the nostrils and face and advise them to avoid exertion and not to blow their nose for a few hours as this may re-start the bleeding.

Internal Bleeding

Internal bleeding can be very difficult to diagnose as the blood loss is not visible. It usually results from direct impact or blunt trauma to the body, although it could develop as a result of certain medical conditions such as perforating ulcers. The main recognition points are:

- History of direct impact or an underlying medical condition.
- There may be pain or tenderness in the area of damage.
- Signs and symptoms of shock may be present (see section 8).

On examination, the skin above the area of damage may become discoloured. This is due to the blood seeping into the upper tissues which will eventually form a bruise.

It is virtually impossible for anyone other than a surgeon to bring internal bleeding under control but simple first aid techniques may at least reduce the bleeding and reduce the speed of deterioration.

- Lay the casualty down in a comfortable position, preferably on their back with the legs slightly raised and keep them still. If the bleeding is in the abdomen, it may be more comfortable for the casualty if the knees are drawn up to the body, thus helping to relax the abdominal muscles.
- Treat the casualty for shock (see section 8).
- If the casualty becomes unconscious, place in the recovery position and be prepared to resuscitate if necessary.
- Call for an ambulance as soon as possible.

Blood-borne Viruses

There are numerous infections which can be spread from person to person by contact with blood and other body fluids, the most well known being Hepatitis B and HIV.

Body fluids other than blood, eg vomit, saliva, sweat, tears, urine, faeces and sputum, are of very minimal risk unless containing blood. You need to take care with these, as the presence of blood is not always visible.

Blood-borne viruses are unlikely to infect a first-aider who acts hygienically. Remember, contamination with these usually occurs accidentally, for example through "sharps" (needles, broken glass). Avoid getting body fluids in open wounds, abrasions, eyes, nose or mouth, and take care if you have a skin condition like eczema.

- Always treat blood and body fluids with caution.
- Ensure that any small cuts or open wounds on your own hands are covered with adhesive dressings.
- If a wound is small and needs cleaning with fresh tap water or a moist cleansing wipe, let the casualty do this themselves.
- Wear protective gloves (latex, vinyl, polythene, etc). Be particularly careful when removing the gloves.

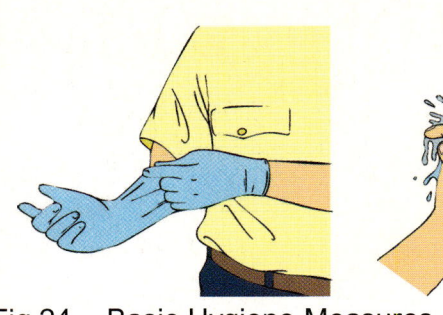

Fig.24. Basic Hygiene Measures

- Use eye protection and disposable waterproof apron if splashing is possible.
- Try as far as is practically possible to avoid contact with blood and broken skin.
- Always clean up properly after an accident. Spillages of blood will need to be disinfected One part bleach to ten parts cold water is a useful guide.
- When you have finished at the scene of an accident, wash your hands.

If a first-aider becomes contaminated with blood:

- wash the area with soap and water
- wash any wound with cold water and encourage it to bleed
- rinse any splashes to eyes, nose or mouth with plenty of tap water, but don't swallow it
- report it and get fast medical help - don't delay.

Test Your Knowledge

1) List 4 things you should do to protect yourself and a casualty from cross-infection, when treating an open wound:

    1 ....
    2 ....
    3 ....
    4 ....

2) Identify 4 main aims when treating someone with severe external bleeding:

    1 ....
    2 ....
    3 ....
    4 ....

3) Describe the correct positioning of casualties who are suffering from the following:

    a) Conscious - suspected angina ....
    b) Unconscious - puncture wound to right chest wall ....
    c) Unconscious - bleeding from the left ear ....
    d) Conscious - severe nose bleed ....
    e) Epilepsy - after the convulsions have ceased ....
    f) Asthma attack - ....

5) Name 3 types of bleeding from an open wound. (Place in order of severity and describe.)

    i ....
    ii ....
    iii ....

Shock

Shock is a very common condition which in some cases can be life-threatening. A good knowledge and understanding of the condition is essential for all appointed persons.

There are many different types of shock, each with their own individual causes and effects. Appointed persons in the workplace may encounter three types.

- Nervous Shock (Neurogenic)
- True Shock (Hypovolaemic)
- Allergic Shock (Anaphylactic)

Nervous Shock

> This is the body's physical reaction to an overwhelming emotional stimulus.

In the early stages only reassurance is usually required but if the condition deteriorates the casualty may faint (see section 9).

In some cases, a casualty in nervous shock may begin to panic and over-react to the situation, becoming what most people would term as 'hysterical'. This panic attack may cause palpitations, trembling, sweating, crying and screaming.

Treatment

- Move the casualty to a quiet place and give lots of reassurance.
- If the casualty has a full panic attack, continue to provide reassurance but be firm and do not over-sympathise with them.
- If the casualty begins to hyperventilate, treat accordingly (see appendix G).
- Stay with the casualty until they have recovered, and advise them to consult with their doctor.
- **X** DO NOT become aggressive, and slap the casualty's face or restrain them, as this could make them worse.

True Shock
Low (hypo) volume (vol) of blood (aemic).

> This is defined as a reduction in the volume and pressure of circulating blood.

Blood exerts a certain pressure inside all blood vessels. This keeps the vessels open in their tube shape. If blood or plasma is lost from the blood vessels, the inside pressure will begin to fall and eventually the vessels may collapse. This reduces the blood and oxygen supply to the vital organs.

A reduction in blood pressure stimulating the onset of true shock can be caused by:

- blood loss;
- plasma loss from burns;
- water loss from dehydration (remember, 95% of plasma is water);
- insufficient pumping of the heart muscle, e.g. during a heart attack.

The body's reaction to a fall in blood pressure is to divert blood from less important areas of the body such as the arms, legs, skin and intestines to the most important areas in the centre of the body such as the heart muscle, brain, lung tissues and other vital organs. This natural body defence mechanism is responsible for producing most of the signs and symptoms of shock. The more the blood pressure falls, the more pronounced the signs and symptoms become.

Recognition

- The skin will become pale and feel cold to the touch, due to the warm, red blood pulling away. Cyanosis (blueness) may develop at the extremities.
- Cold skin may stimulate the casualty to shiver in an attempt to generate heat. This is not good, as the unwanted muscular activity will burn off more vital oxygen and stimulate blood flow to the limbs and main muscles, away from the vital organs.
- The casualty will begin to sweat. The nervous stimulus which controls the defence mechanism also controls the body's sweating mechanism. A cold sweat is an unwanted side effect of shock, as it means more fluid loss.
- The casualty may feel dizzy or faint. This is due to the oxygen reduction in the brain.
- The casualty may feel nauseous or may actually vomit. This feeling is often made

worse if the casualty has recently eaten or has consumed alcohol.

- The casualty may feel weak and lethargic. This is caused by a lack of oxygen and glucose (sugar) to the main muscles.
- The casualty may feel thirsty. To conserve body fluid, the salivary glands stop functioning and the mouth becomes dry. Many people have suffered this symptom as a result of dehydration, especially a hangover.
- The pulse rate will increase and gradually become weaker. To try and increase blood pressure, the heart will beat faster but as the pressure inside the arteries continues to fall, so will the amount of blood passing through them.
- The breathing rate will increase in an attempt to saturate the remaining blood with as much oxygen as possible. As it increases in speed, it becomes weak and shallow. In the later stages the casualty may begin to gasp for air.

The condition of shock is aggravated or made worse by:

- An abnormal body temperature, e.g. by becoming too warm or too cold.
- An upright posture (as gravity pulls blood into the legs, away from the vital organs).
- Eating and drinking. This may make the nausea worse and if the casualty becomes unconscious, it could contribute to vomiting.
- Smoking. Every inhalation of a cigarette puts hundreds of toxins into the blood stream which will reach the brain and other organs in just a few seconds.

Treatment

The treatment of true shock is very simple and can be very effective.

- Identify and, if possible, treat the underlying cause, e.g. control any bleeding or cool down a burn.
- Lay the casualty down. This stops blood pulling into the legs and increases blood flow to the brain and other vital organs.
- Elevate their legs (if injuries allow). This again helps divert blood from the legs to the vital organs.
- Maintain a normal body temperature. Wrap the casualty in a coat or blanket to help retain their natural body heat and prevent shivering.
- Keep the airway open and clear, and loosen any tight or restrictive clothing.
- Reassure the casualty throughout.
- Always call for an ambulance if a casualty should develop true shock.
- If the casualty becomes unconscious, place into the recovery position and monitor breathing and circulation.

X Do not give the casualty anything to eat or drink (including alcohol) as this may cause vomiting and may interfere with any future hospital treatments.

X Do not over-heat the casualty as this will stimulate blood flow to the extremities in an attempt to lose unwanted body heat.

X Do not allow the casualty to smoke.

Allergic Shock

This is a major allergic reaction within the body. It can be a very serious condition and, in extreme cases, life-threatening.

Test Your Knowledge

1) Give 4 measures you should take to treat a casualty you think is suffering from shock:

   i ....
   ii ....
   iii ....
   iv ....

2) State the effect that shock is likely to have on the following:

   i   Pulse ....
   ii   Breathing ....
   iii Skin ....
   iv   How the casualty feels ....

Head Injuries

Although preventable, injuries to the head are common in many working environments and in some cases they can be very serious.

The brain is situated inside the skull for protection, and as we have already seen, it is one of the most important organs of the body. The function of the brain is to control and co-ordinate the majority of body functions. Injuries to the head can cause temporary or permanent damage to the brain which can have a widespread and sometimes life-threatening effect.

Concussion

This is a temporary and reversible disturbance of the brain's normal function. It occurs when the brain moves or 'shakes' inside the skull and is usually caused by a blow to the head or jaw.

Recognition

Concussion can occur without causing unconsciousness, or in some cases the duration of unconsciousness may have been so brief that the casualty cannot remember the initial accident.

- History of a blow to, or shaking of, the head.
- There may be some disturbance in normal vision.
- The casualty may feel nauseous or may vomit.
- Possible dizziness or giddiness.
- The casualty may complain of a headache.
- There may be a partial loss of memory, particularly of the events immediately before the accident.
- Possible unconsciousness, usually of short duration

Treatment

In most cases, the treatment of concussion only involves rest and monitoring the casualty for any deterioration (as a reversible condition it should go away on its own). In all cases, however, the casualty must be advised to see their doctor after work or if any symptoms are persistent or become worse.

- Keep the casualty at rest and reassure them.
- If necessary, carry out the treatment for the unconscious casualty and call for an ambulance.
- If there is a lump or bump developing on the head, apply a cold compress to reduce swelling.
- Monitor the casualty for signs and symptoms which may indicate cerebral compression, even if the casualty has apparently recovered.
- If the casualty suffered unconsciousness, even for a short period, arrange for them to be taken to hospital for further examination and observation.
- If any signs or symptoms are still present, or the casualty feels at all unwell, arrange for them to be taken to hospital for further examination and observation.
- If all signs and all symptoms have gone, the casualty may return to work but keep an eye on them and tell them to report back to you if any symptoms recur or they begin to feel unwell. Remember though, the casualty must still be advised to see their doctor after work.

X DO NOT let the casualty lie down or sleep in the first aid or rest room following concussion. It is much harder to spot deterioration in the condition when the casualty is asleep. If the casualty is unable to sit up due to the severity of the concussion, they should go to hospital immediately.

Compression of the Brain

This is due to a build up of pressure within the skull. The pressure is exerted onto the brain and seriously interferes with its ability to control and co-ordinate the functions of the body. It can result in permanent damage to the brain.

Pressure can build up inside the skull for a variety of reasons including medical conditions such as tumours, injuries such as bleeding from blood vessels inside the skull or depressed fractures of the skull.

The onset of compression is not always sudden, and it can develop some hours or even days after a head injury. This is why observations on a casualty who has suffered concussion are so important.

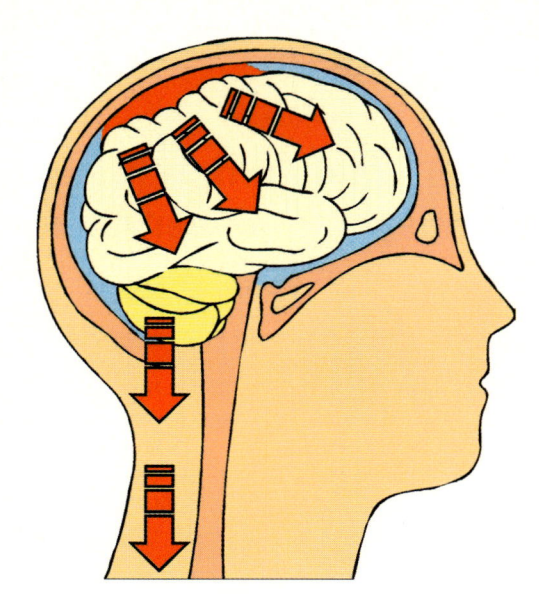

Fig.25. Compression Injury

Recognition

As the condition develops, the signs and symptoms become more and more pronounced.

- History of an unusual, persistent headache or history of impact to the head.
- In the initial stages, the signs and symptoms of concussion may be present.
- As the compression develops, the casualty's level of response will deteriorate. In most cases this will result in unconsciousness.
- While the casualty remains conscious, a weakness or paralysis of one side of the body may develop.
- Breathing may become laboured, noisy and irregular.
- The pulse rate may slow down and become strong and irregular.
- The pupils may be different sizes, and their reaction to light may become slow or absent.
- The casualty's skin temperature may rise, and his face may become flushed and warm to the touch. This is due to a rise in blood pressure.

Treatment

There is nothing that the appointed person can do to release the pressure building up inside the skull so treatment revolves around A.B.C.

- If the casualty is conscious, place and support them in a comfortable position, preferably with the head and shoulders slightly raised.
- Treat any other injuries, such as bleeding from a scalp wound.
- If the casualty is unconscious, place in recovery position and ensure the airway remains open and clear.
- Carry out resuscitation if necessary.
- Call for an ambulance as soon as possible.

Spinal/neck/skull injuries

Use the jaw thrust to maintain an airway in these casualties, unless they are vomiting or you need to leave them.

- Kneel behind the casualty's head.
- Place your hands on each side of the head with your fingertips at the angles of the jaw.
- Gently lift the jaw to open the airway.
- Take care not to tilt the casualty's head.

If vomiting or unconscious and you need to leave the casualty, use a recovery position:

- "Normal" recovery position if you are alone.
- If you have one helper, one person steadies the head and second person turns the casualty.
- If you have two helpers, one person steadies the head and the second turns the casualty and the third helps to keep the back in alignment with the head.
- If you have three or more helpers, use the log roll technique – remove spectacles and bulky objects in pockets.

Don't forget to "read the accident" – if there is a history of force to the body of any sort, always suspect spinal injuries.

Bleeding from the Scalp

The scalp has a very good blood supply which helps in the body's heat control mechanism. Although high in number, the blood vessels in the scalp are relatively small and therefore controlling bleeding is usually easy.

Treatment

- Rest and reassure the casualty.
- Examine the wound for any obvious embedded object.
- Control the bleeding with gentle pressure, using a sterile wound dressing.
- If the wound is large or the bleeding will not stop, arrange for them to be taken to hospital for further treatment.
- Monitor for signs of concussion and treat accordingly.

General Illness at Work

As an appointed person, you may find that you spend just as much time dealing with people who don't feel well as you do dealing with people who have injuries.

It is important that the appointed person is aware of the actions which should be taken when presented with illnesses at work, remembering that the ill person needs to be safe as a result of your treatment.

Serious medical conditions which can come on suddenly and may constitute a medical emergency such as asthma, heart conditions, stroke, diabetes and epilepsy are covered in the appendix of this manual.

Common, and more minor, illnesses which may occur at work include headache, toothache, earache, stomach-ache/nausea and cold/influenza.

Many common ailments may be relieved by proprietary drugs which can be bought over the counter from a chemist or other outlet. The decision to take these medicines is the responsibility of the person suffering the ailment and is outside the responsibility of the appointed person. **It is stressed that under no circumstances should an appointed person advise an ill person to take, or actually dispense, any medication whatsoever at work.** This could land you and your company in big trouble!

In some cases of illness at work, the person may have suffered from the illness before, and may even be taking medication prescribed by their doctor. If this is the case, the ill person will know when, and how, to take such medication.

General Points when Dealing with Illness at Work

It must be remembered that people at work are of adult age, and therefore capable of making decisions for themselves with regard to their condition and what action should be taken.

- An appointed person is not expected to be able to make a true diagnosis of the underlying illness (this is a doctor's job). However, the appointed person is expected to be able to make a common-sense decision about their overall condition and what action should be taken next.

- If possible, deal with the person in a quiet, private area such as the first-aid room.

- Always listen carefully and sympathetically to any history or symptoms which the person tells you.

- Whether you have an idea or not of what may be the cause of the problem, never have any doubt about someone who is ill at work. Get qualified medical help rather than hope for the best.

- In many cases, the only treatment that an appointed person can give for an illness is advice.

  - If the person feels well enough to return to work, and at their request, they may do so. However, it is good practice for the appointed person to look in on the person from time to time throughout the day to check on their condition. The casualty should always be advised to see their doctor should the condition persist or worsen.

  - If, in their own opinion, the person is too ill to return to work, at their request they may wish to go home. If this is the case, the appointed person should ensure that the chosen method of transportation home will be safe, bearing in mind their illness. For example, a casualty who is having bad migraine which is causing disturbances in their vision and concentration should not be allowed to drive themselves home.

  - If any person is too ill to continue work, they are ill enough to warrant seeing their doctor. Bearing this in mind, the appointed person should always advise the casualty to see their doctor as soon as possible. If they don't take your advice, that is their decision.

- If the nature of the illness is such that it could spread from person to person (communicable), the casualty should not be allowed to continue work and should be advised to see their doctor immediately. If they remain at work, it could put other members of staff at risk and will not allow for rest, which is an important factor in their recovery. Examples of common communicable illness are influenza, and diarrhoea/vomiting.

- If a person is unable to continue work due to an illness, inform their supervisor or manager at the earliest possible opportunity.

- It is advisable that all occurrences of illness at work are formally recorded.
  - It will confirm that the illness was dealt with correctly by the appointed person and provide a written record of any advice which was given.
  - It will allow management to review occurrences of illness at work and evaluate the potential of the working environment causing or contributing towards the illness.

The Particular Needs of Female Colleagues

There are a few conditions which could develop at work which are unique to female members of staff. Two common conditions are painful periods (dysmenorrhoea) and problems during pregnancy.

- It is often best that a female appointed person deals with this nature of problem.

- Always be discreet, offering privacy and rest.
- The person themselves are usually the best judge of their needs, so listen to them carefully.
- If there is any suspicion that the discomfort being experienced is not usual or normal, seek further medical aid.

Mental Distress

If you notice unusual behaviour such as irritability or aggression, or bouts of uncontrollable weeping, it may be an indication of mental distress.

Your colleague needs to seek medical help and may need quietness, support, time and encouragement to get help.

If you are worried about your colleague, you may need to arrange for them to go to hospital. Make sure that somebody else drives you there.

Test Your Knowledge

1) Name six signs or symptoms which could help you in your diagnosis of any illness/injury:

i ....
ii ....
iii ....
iv ....
v ....
vi ....

Moving a Casualty

Under certain circumstances, a casualty may have to be moved. It is important that an appointed person has a good understanding of when this may be necessary and how to do it safely.

Appointed persons should never attempt to move or lift a casualty, except in the most extreme of emergencies. Where there is no danger at the scene of the accident to the casualty or appointed person, the casualty should remain where they are until expert help arrives.

If a workplace has difficult or restricted access, the risk assessment should take this into consideration and, where necessary, provide mechanical aids for the lifting and movement of injured people, such as a 'carry chair'. Additional training will be required for anyone responsible for using such specialised equipment.

There are four main situations that can be regarded as true emergencies and which may require a casualty to be immediately removed from danger. In such cases, the rescuers must consider the risks to themselves - remember, do not become a casualty yourself!

- Danger from a collapsing building or falling object.
- An area that is on fire or filling with smoke or other harmful gases and fumes.
- In water where the casualty is in danger of drowning.
- Danger from explosion or firearms.

In an emergency, and where the manual handling of injured people is necessary, the following guidelines should be adhered to:

- **Avoid lifting**
  - whenever possible, do not lift;
  - encourage people to help themselves;
  - make use of available equipment and lifting aids.

- **If lifting is unavoidable:**
  - assess the task:
    - what are you going to do?
    - why is it necessary?
    - what are the difficulties and constraints?
  - assess the casualty:
    - how heavy are they?
    - what is their ability with regard to communication and helping themselves?
    - what physical and behavioural constraints are there, including injuries?
  - the environment:
    - location and conditions
    - the distance and route to be travelled
    - availability of help and specialised equipment
  - yourself:
    - level of skill
    - fitness and ability
    - clothing

Making the Lift

- Get someone to help you if possible - 'many hands make light work'.
- Keep the weight as close to yourself as possible.
- Keep the feet placed a shoulder width apart to ensure good balance.
- Bend the knees and keep the back straight.
- Avoid twisting and stooping.
- Raise your head as you start to lift.
- Lift with the power of the leg muscles, not the back.

Transportation Methods

The Human Crutch Method

This method can be used if the casualty is conscious and able to walk with some assistance.

- If available, give the casualty a walking aid.
- Stand on the weakest or injured side of the casualty.

- Pass the casualty's arm around your neck and grasp their hand or wrist with your hand.
- Place your other arm around the casualty's waist and grasp hold of their belt or clothing for extra support.
- Taking small steps, move off with the inside foot. Allow the pace to be governed by the casualty.
- Offer continual encouragement and reassurance to the casualty.

The Drag Method

This method should only be used in an emergency, to move a casualty who is unconscious or unable to walk. The method described should not be used if there are injuries to the head or neck or back (although if the casualty is unconscious, this may be difficult to determine).

- Squat behind the casualty and assist them to sit up with their arms crossed over their chest.
- Place your arms under the casualty's armpits and grasp their wrists.
- Carefully, whilst squat walking backwards, drag the casualty clear.

If the casualty is wearing a coat or jacket, it may be easier to move them as follows:

- Unbutton the coat or jacket.
- Pull the jacket up under the head.
- grasp the jacket under the casualty's shoulders and gently drag them clear.

Carry Chairs

These chairs are used in many shops, schools, hotels and other places of work. They are designed to allow for the evacuation of casualties (or disabled people) up or down stairs and along corridors. Most carry chairs have two or four wheels which makes the movement along flat surfaces much easier. They also have carrying handles for use when going up or down stairs.

Where carry chairs are provided, appropriate training must be given in their use.

- Unfold the chair and test its safety by pressing down on the seat.
- Sit the casualty in the chair and secure the safety harness over the casualty's arms.
- Place the casualty's feet on the foot bar.
- Always support the back of the chair to prevent it from tipping backward.

Moving (one appointed person)

- Reassure the casualty and explain what you are going to do.
- If the chair has four wheels, simply push it forward at a controlled speed.
- If the chair has only two rear wheels, carefully tip the chair back and push it forward at a controlled speed, continually reassuring the casualty.

X Do not pull the chair.

Down stairs (only with help)

A casualty who is being moved up or down stairs in a carry chair will feel very insecure and anxious; therefore, reassure them throughout the procedure.

- Stand behind the chair, facing down the stairs. The helper should stand a few steps down, facing the chair.
- Gently tip the chair back and the helper should now firmly grasp the carrying handles on the foot bar.
- On the command of the helper, the chair is lifted.
- The helper should control the pace of the journey down the stairs, step by step.

Up Stairs

- Reverse the procedure.

Test Your Knowledge

1) Give three principles of safe moving:

   i ....
   ii ....
   iii ....

After an Accident at Work

In addition to providing treatments, the appointed person is also responsible for dealing with the 'aftermath' of an accident at work.

There are three tasks which must be performed immediately after an accident at work:

1. Tidying up.
2. Recording details of the accident and any treatments given.
3. Re-stocking the first aid box.

Tidying Up

(As HIV and Hepatitis B Virus stay active for considerable periods of time in dried blood, it is important for employees to be aware of their company's code of practice for dealing with spillages, etc.)

There are two types of waste material which may be produced when dealing with a casualty at work, routine waste and clinical waste.

Routine Waste

This relates to any paper or wrapping from first aid equipment which has been used. If it is uncontaminated, it should simply be put into the normal waste bin.

Clinical Waste

This relates to any items contaminated by the casualty's blood, vomit, saliva or urine. It is improper and potentially unsafe to put this type of waste into the normal bin as it may contain a considerable risk of biological hazard. Clinical waste requires specific management.

- Wear disposable gloves, and apron to protect your clothing.
- If there is spillage of blood, vomit or urine on the floor, it should be disinfected with a suitable solution. There are many proprietary brands of disinfection solution available from medical wholesalers and high street shops. It is often best to use a powdered form of disinfectant rather than a liquid as this will soak up the spillage, not spread it further.

When using disinfectant solution, always follow the advice on the container and, if necessary, wear protective goggles.

- Contaminated dressings, material and paper packets should be carefully placed into a polythene bag. Remember to put your gloves and apron into the bag before sealing it up.
- Yellow bags, as used in first aid-rooms, should be disposed of by incineration. This must be performed in a proper clinical incinerator and not on a makeshift bonfire in the company car park.

There are two possible ways of ensuring that it is dealt with correctly:

- If available at work, have the bag put into the sanitary towel waste bin in the ladies toilet. Contract cleaners will now remove the clinical waste from the premises in the correct manner and ensure its safe incineration.
- Contact your Council or local authority who usually offer a collection service for this type of low-grade, small-quantity biological waste.

(As HIV and Hepatitis B Virus stay active for considerable periods of time in dried blood, it is important for employees to be aware of their company's code of practice for dealing with spillages, etc.)

Recording Details

It is a legal requirement that details of all accidents in the workplace are recorded in an appropriate manner (this even includes accidents where no one was injured). In many cases, this simply involves filling in the accident book or other suitable in-house form which your company may provide.

The appointed person must be able to maintain a simple, factual record of any and all treatments which they have administered at work (even if the only treatment possible was advice to the casualty).

Good record keeping provides a detailed and accurate account of all details relating to the accident and injuries sustained, and this is necessary for many reasons:

- it will allow the employer to evaluate the effectiveness of existing safety policies and procedures;

- it may indicate to the employer the need for new safety policies and procedures (the employer cannot take steps to prevent further accidents and injuries happening if they are unaware of their initial occurrence);
- it may be used as documentary evidence in any legal proceedings concerning compensation, or negligence by the employer or employee.

General Points on Recording and Reporting Accidents

- It is essential that the appointed person is familiar with the location of documents used in their own workplace and how to complete them correctly.
- As an absolute minimum, the following details should always be recorded:
  - full name and address of the person who suffered an accident;
  - their occupation;
  - the date when the entry was made;
- the date and time of the accident;
- the place and circumstances of the accident, stating clearly the work process which was being performed at the time of the accident;
- details of any injuries suffered and any treatment given;
- signature of the person making the entry and their address.
- All details should be written in pen and should be neat and legible.
- Be specific with details relating to the location of injuries, for example '1cm cut to middle finger of left hand' is much more specific than 'cut finger'.
- If ever in doubt about how to record any details, seek the advice of your manager or supervisor.
- If a casualty is so bad that they have to go to their doctor or hospital, inform your manager or supervisor verbally as soon as possible. In some cases, further reporting of the accident to an enforcing authority may be necessary under RIDDOR Regulations (see section 1).

Test Your Knowledge

1) As a "First Aid at Work" designated appointed person, you may have to maintain records:

   a) What records are required to be kept by law? ....

   b) Give 2 reasons why it is important to keep records:

      i ....

      ii ....

2) After you have cleaned an area where blood has been spilled, what solution of bleach to water do you use?

   .... part/s bleach to .... part/s water

3) Which of the following does not need reporting under RIDDOR (please tick one answer):

   a) Spinal fracture
   b) An injury that involved the employee being off work for four days
   c) A car accident on the way to work resulting in the death of an employee
   d) A doctor reports to the employer that an employee has a work-related disease of a contagious nature

First-Aid Equipment

Maintaining a suitable and adequate supply of first-aid equipment, based on the needs of the particular workplace, is essential.

Information in this section is taken from the Health and Safety (First-Aid) Regulations 1981 and the accompanying Approved Code of Practice and Guidance

The Health and Safety (First-Aid) Regulations 1981 require every employer to:

"...ensure that there are provided, such equipment and facilities as are adequate and appropriate in the circumstances for enabling first aid to be rendered to his employees if they are injured or become ill at work".

How much first-aid provision an employer has to make depends on the circumstances in each workplace. No fixed level exists, but each employer needs to assess what facilities (and personnel) are appropriate.

When the assessment of first-aid requirements has been completed, the employer should provide the materials, equipment and facilities needed to ensure that the level of cover identified as necessary will be available to employees at all relevant times. This will include ensuring that first-aid equipment, suitably marked and easily accessible, is available in all places where working conditions require it.

First-Aid Containers

The minimum level of first-aid equipment is a suitably stocked and properly identified first-aid container. Every employer should provide for each work site at least one first-aid container, supplied with a sufficient quantity of first-aid materials suitable for the particular circumstances.

First-aid containers should be easily accessible and placed, if possible, near to hand-washing facilities. Employers assessing the need for first-aid provision on large sites should consider providing more than one first-aid container. The container should protect the equipment from dust and damp and should only be stocked with items useful for giving first aid.

Tablets and medications should not be kept, nor should equipment for which the appointed person has not been trained in its use.

The container must be identified by a white cross on a green background.

There is no mandatory list of items that should be included in a first-aid container but, as a guide, where no special risk arises in the workplace, a minimum stock of first-aid items would normally be:

- a leaflet giving general guidance on first aid;
- twenty individually wrapped sterile adhesive dressings in assorted sizes. These should be appropriate to the type of work (dressings may be of a detectable type for food handlers);
- two sterile eye pads;
- four individually wrapped triangular bandages (preferably sterile);
- six safety pins;
- six medium-sized individually wrapped sterile unmedicated wound dressings - approximately 12cm x 12cm;
- two large-sized individually wrapped sterile unmedicated wound dressings - approximately 18cm x 18cm;
- one pair of disposable gloves.

This is a suggested contents list only; equivalent but different items will be considered acceptable.

The contents of first-aid containers should be checked at least once a week, and should be re-stocked as soon as possible after use. Sufficient supplies should be held in a back-up stock on site.

Care should be taken to discard items safely after the expiry date has passed.

Additional First-Aid Equipment

The assessment may conclude that there is a need for additional materials and equipment: for example, resuscitation barrier devices, scissors, adhesive tape, disposable aprons and individually wrapped moist wipes. These may be kept in the first-aid container if there is room, but they may be stored separately as long as they are available for use if required.

In particular circumstances, the assessment may identify a need for items such as protective equipment, in case, for example, appointed persons have to enter dangerous atmospheres; or blankets to protect casualties from the elements. These additional items should be securely stored near the first-aid container, in the first-aid room or in the hazard area, as appropriate. It is important that access to these items is restricted to people trained in their use.

Where mains tap water is not readily available for eye irrigation, at least a litre of sterile water or sterile normal saline (0.9%) in sealed, disposable containers should be provided. Once the seal has been broken, the contents should not be kept for re-use. The container should not be used after the expiry date.

Travelling First-Aid Kits

First-aid kits for travelling workers would typically contain:

- a leaflet giving general guidance on first aid;
- six individually wrapped sterile adhesive dressings;
- one large sterile unmedicated dressing - approximately 18cm x 18cm;
- two triangular bandages;
- two safety pins;
- individually wrapped moist cleansing wipes;
- one pair of disposable gloves.

This is a suggested contents list only; equivalent but different items will be considered acceptable. As with first-aid containers, the contents of kits should be kept stocked from the back-up stock at the home site.

First-Aid Rooms

Employers should provide a suitable first-aid room or rooms where the assessment of first-aid needs identifies this as necessary. The first-aid room should contain essential first-aid facilities and equipment, be easily accessible to stretchers and be clearly signposted and identified by white lettering or symbols on a green background. If possible, the room should be reserved exclusively for giving first aid.

A first-aid room will usually be necessary in establishments with high risks, such as shipbuilding firms, chemical industries or large construction sites and in larger premises at a distance from medical services. A designated person should be given responsibility for the room.

To be effective, first-aid rooms should:

- be large enough to hold a couch, with enough space at each side for people to work, a desk, a chair and any necessary additional equipment;
- have washable surfaces and adequate heating, ventilation and lighting;
- be kept clean, tidy, accessible and available for use at all times when employees are at work;
- be positioned as near as possible to a point of access for transport to hospital;
- display a notice on the door advising of the names, locations and, if appropriate, telephone extensions of appointed persons and how to contact them.

Typical examples of the facilities and equipment a first-aid room may contain are:

- a sink with hot and cold running water;
- drinking water and disposable cups;
- soap and paper towels;
- a store for first-aid materials;
- an adequate supply of first-aid materials, similar in type to those kept in the first-aid container. Remember, an appointed person should only use equipment in which they have been trained;
- foot-operated refuse containers, lined with yellow clinical waste bags or a container suitable for the safe disposal of clinical waste;
- a couch with waterproof protection and clean pillows and blankets;
- a chair;
- a telephone or other communication equipment;
- a record book for recording incidents where first aid has been given.

If the first-aid room cannot be reserved exclusively for giving first aid, employers need to take care that the first-aid facilities can be made available quickly if necessary. For example, they should consider the implications of whether:

- the activities usually carried out in the room can be stopped immediately in an emergency;
- the furnishings and equipment can be moved easily and quickly to a position that will not interfere with giving first aid;
- the storage arrangements for first-aid furnishings and equipment allow them to be made quickly available when necessary.

> The contents of the first-aid room should be checked on a regular basis, e.g. once a week and re-stocked as soon as possible. Date-expired items should be carefully discarded.

Re-supply of First-Aid Equipment

It is important that appointed persons familiarise themselves with the already-established procedure for the re-supply of first-aid equipment in their workplace.

If there is no such procedure in place, liaise with the employer and formulate one.

There are many possible sources for the purchase and re-supply of first-aid materials and equipment. The approved training organisation who ran your first aid course may sell first-aid equipment as a part of their service, or at least they may be able to recommend a potential source of purchase. Alternatively, look in your local business telephone directory under 'First-Aid Equipment Suppliers'.

Test Your Knowledge

1) Delete from the following the items which should not be found in a first aid box which conforms to Health & Safety guidelines:

　　a) scissors　　　b) safety pins　　　c) antiseptic cream　　　d) eye pads

　　e) eye bath　　　f) medium dressings　　　g) adhesive dressings　　　h) extra large dressings

　　i) tweezers　　　j) sterile triangulars　　　k) guidance leaflet　　　l) large dressings

Index

A B C of First Aid	2.4	First-Aid Rooms	13.2
Abdominal Thrust	4.2	Head Injuries	9.1
Accidents at Work	12.1	Health & Safety – Legislation	1.1
Accident Reporting	12.1	Human Crutch	11.1
Adhesive Dressings	7.1	Illness at Work	10.1
Aim of First Aid Treatment	2.2	Indirect Pressure	7.3
Allergic Shock	8.2	Impalement	7.5
Ambulance – Calling For	5.3	Infection – Signs & Symptoms	7.1
Amputations	7.5	Internal Bleeding	7.6
Arterial Bleeding	7.1	Major Wounds	7.1
Artificial Ventilation	3.1	Medic Alert	6.4
Assessment of a Situation	2.1	Mental Stress	10.2
Back slaps	4.2	Minor Wounds	7.1
Bleeding – Types	7.1	Moving a Casualty	11.1
Bleeding Limbs	7.5	Nervous Shock	8.1
Bleeding Scalp	7.5	Nosebleed	7.6
Bleeding from the Scalp	9.2	Observations to Record	6.6
Bleeding Palm	7.5	Opening the Airway	5.2
Blood Borne Viruses	7.6	Pressure Points	7.3
Calling for an Ambulance	2.5	Preventing a Condition Worsening	2.3
Non-Breathing Casualty	5.3	Record Keeping	12.1
Capillary Bleeding	7.1	Recording Accidents	12.1
Carry Chairs	11.2	Recovery Position	6.4
Chest Compressions	3.2	Rescue Breathing	3.1
Choking	4.1	Responsibilities of an Appointed Person	2.1
Clinical Waste	12.1	Re-supply of First-Aid Equipment	13.3
Compression	9.1	Resuscitation	3.1
Concussion	9.1	Resuscitation Flow Chart	3.4
Cross Infection	7.6	Saving Life	2.3
Diagnosis	2.1	Shock	8.1
Direct Pressure	7.2	Stoppage of Circulation	3.2
Disposal of a Casualty	2.4	Stoppage of Breathing	3.1
Disposal of Waste	12.1	Tablets and Medicines	13.1
Dragging a Casualty	11.2	Travelling First-Aid Kits	13.2
Dressings	7.2	Unconsciousness	6.1
Embedded Objects	7.4	common causes	6.1
Emergency Diagnosis	5.1	examination/treatment	6.2
Fainting	6.1	Venous Bleeding	7.1
Female Colleagues	10.2	Waste	12.1
First-Aid Containers	13.1	Wounds and Bleeding	7.1
First-Aid Equipment	13.1		

PAGE I • 1

For Your Notes

For Your Notes

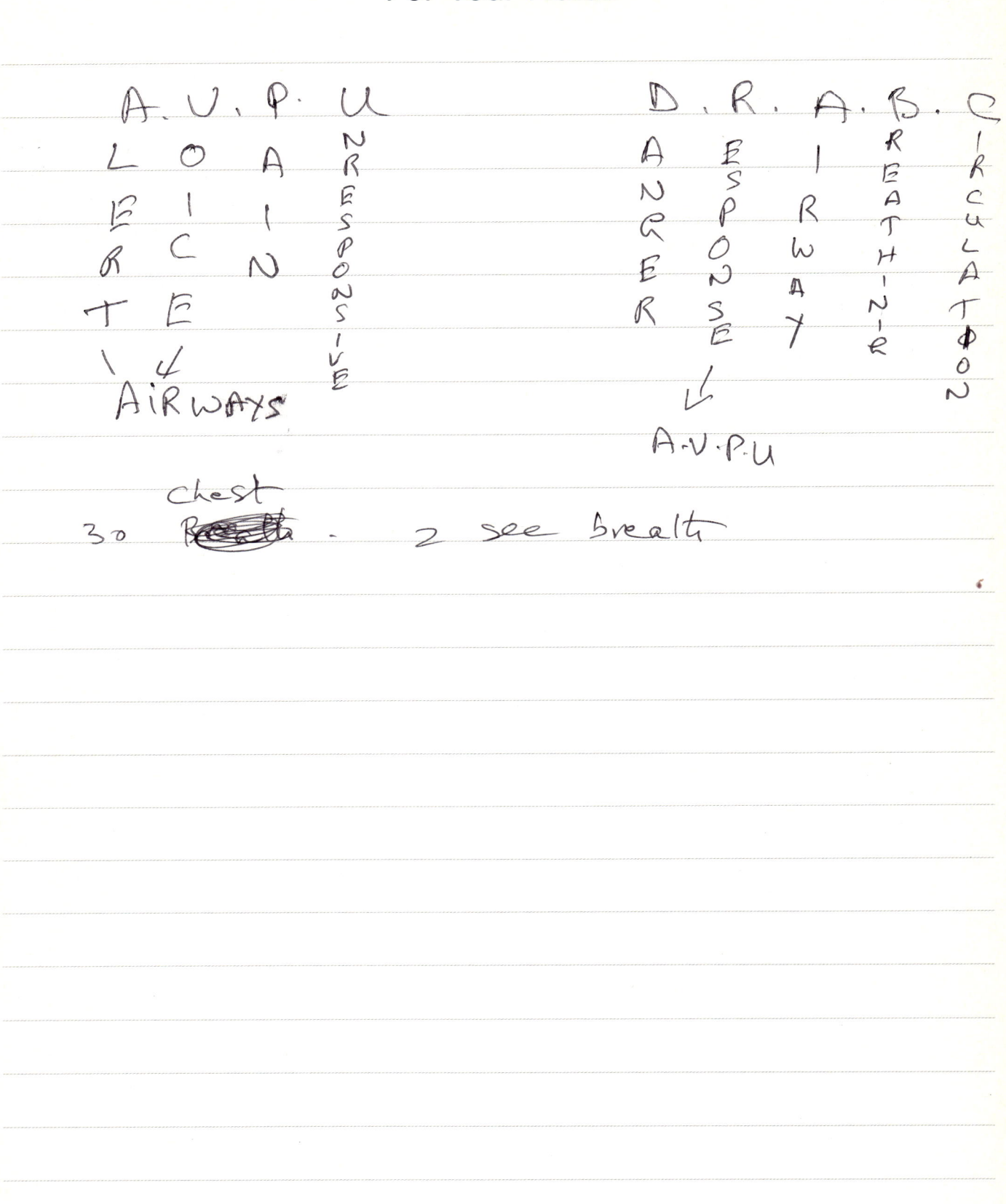

A.V.P.U
- **A**lert
- **V**oice
- **P**ain
- **U**nresponsive

Airways

D.R.A.B.C
- **D**anger
- **R**esponse
- **A**irway
- **B**reathing
- **C**irculation

↓
A.V.P.U

30 chest [scribble] · 2 see breath